Common Eye Diseases and their Ma

Springer
London
Berlin
Heidelberg
New York
Barcelona
Hong Kong
Milan
Paris
Santa Clara
Singapore
Tokyo

N.R. Galloway and W.M.K. Amoaku

Common Eye Diseases and their Management

2nd Edition

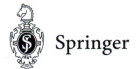

Springer

Nicholas Robert Galloway, MD, FRCS, FRCOphth
Winfried Mawutor Kwaku Amoaku, FRCS, FRCOphth, PhD
Directorate of Ophthalmology, B Floor, South Block, Queen's Medical Centre, University Hospital NHS Trust, Nottingham, NG7 2UH

ISBN 3-540-1-85233-050-3 (2nd Edition) Springer-Verlag London Berlin Heidelberg
ISBN 3-540-13659-2 (1st Edition) Springer-Verlag Berlin Heidelberg New York

British Library Cataloguing in Publication Data
Galloway, N. R. (Nicholas R.)
    Common eye diseases and their management. – 2nd ed.
    1. Eye – Diseases
    I. Title   II. Amoaku, Winfried Manutor Kwaku
    614.7
    ISBN 1852330503

Library of Congress Cataloging-in-Publication Data
Galloway, N. R.
    Common eye diseases and their management / N. R. Galloway and
    W. M. K. Amoaku. – 2nd ed.
        p.   cm.
    Includes bibliographical references and index.
    ISBN 1–85233–050–3 (pbk. :;alk. paper)
    1. Eye–Diseases.   I. Amoaku, W. M. K. (Winfried Mawutor Kwaku),
    1953– .   II. Title.
    [DNLM: 1. Eye Diseases.   WW 140G174c 1999]
    RE46.G34   1999
    617.7–dc21
    for Library of Congress   98–26295

1st Edition published in 1985

Typeset by EXPO Holdings, Kuala Lumpur
Printed and bound at Kyodo Printing Co (S'pore) Pte Ltd, Singapore 628599
28/3830-543210 Printed on acid-free paper

Preface to Second Edition

Like the first edition, this textbook is intended primarily for medical students but it is also aimed at all those involved in the primary care of eye disease including general practitioners, nurses and optometrists. The need for the primary care practitioner to be well informed about common eye conditions is even more important today than when the first edition was produced. A recent survey from North London has shown that 30% of a sample of the population aged 65 and over are visually impaired in both eyes and a large proportion of those with treatable eye conditions were not in touch with eye services. It is clear that better strategies for managing problems of eyesight need to be set up. One obvious strategy is the improved education of those conducting primary care and it is hoped that this book will contribute to this. For this second edition I am very grateful for the help of my co-author Winfried Amoaku whose personal experience in teaching medical students here in Nottingham has been invaluable. His expertise in the management of macular disease, now a major cause of sensory deprivation in the elderly, is also evident in these chapters.

The format of the book has not changed but some of the chapters have been expanded. For example, there is now a section dealing with the eye complications of AIDS. This problem barely existed at the time of the first edition. Cataract surgery has changed a great deal in this short time and is becoming one of the commonest major surgical procedures to be performed in a hospital. The management of glaucoma has also changed with the introduction of a range of new medications. Our aim has been to keep the original problem oriented layout and to keep it as a book to read rather than a book to look at. There are a number of very good atlases on eye disease and some of these are mentioned in the section at the end on further reading. Although the title of the book is 'Common Eye Diseases' some less common conditions are mentioned and it is hoped that the reader will gain some overall impression of the incidence of different eye diseases.

Acknowledgements

I would like once again to acknowledge the painstaking assistance of my secretary, Mrs A. Padgett. Fortunately, advances in word processing have lightened her burden since the first edition but her help has been none the less invaluable. In this edition most of the original line illustrations and cartoons by Geoffrey Lyth have been retained and once again I would like to express my appreciation of his skill. My thanks are also due to Mrs Karen Hills who typed Mr. Amoaku's chapters as well as those colleagues who have kindly contributed illustrations. Roger Dobbing the production manager from Springer has been very helpful in dealing with numerous problems that have arisen along the way, and finally I would also like to thank again all those who helped with the first edition including those first students in the new Nottingham medical school.

Contents

Section III Problems of the Eye Surgeon

Section I

Introducing the Eye

The Scope of Ophthalmology

Those who regard science as the study of more and more about less and less will find that medicine is no exception to this process of specialisation. It is mainly by the intensive study of minutiae that medical science becomes effective and can lead to the prevention and cure of disease. The eye and its surrounding structures provide us with an ideal terrain for this type of specialisation. The importance of the eye and its function in our daily lives is sometimes underrated, but a consideration of the part played by vision in our consciousness soon makes us realise the value of vision. If we think of dreams, memories, of photographs and of almost anything in our daily existence, it is difficult to express them without visual references. After a little careful consideration of the meaning of blindness, it is easy to sense the rational and irrational fears that our patients present in daily life. In a modern European community the effects of blindness are not so apparent as in former years, and blind people tapping their way around the streets or begging for food are less in evidence to remind us of the deprivation that they suffer. This is due to the effective application of preventive medicine and the efficacy of modern surgical techniques. However, in the western world we have a new and increasing problem relating to the increasing number of elderly people in the population. The problem is that of sensory deprivation due to degenerative disease. Degenerative changes in the eye are now a major cause of blindness and although support services are becoming well developed a cure is not at hand.

The broad and detailed scientific interest in the eye and vision is witnessed by the vast number of journals that are available, possibly more than in any other specialty. There are several hundreds of ophthalmological journals all contributing to the scientific literature of the subject and many now accessible through the Internet or CD-ROM. As an organ of specialisation, the eye has another advantage; it can be seen. Using the slit-lamp microscope it is possible to examine living nerves, including central nervous system tissues and blood vessels, in a manner, which is not possible in other parts of the body without endoscopy and biopsy. So much are the component parts of the eye on display to the clinician that when a patient presents to an eye casualty department with symptoms, the explanation of the symptoms should be made evident by careful examination. Compare this with the vague aches and pains, which present to the gastroenterologist or the neurologist, symptoms which ultimately resolve without any cause being found for them. The student or newly qualified doctor must be warned that if the patient presents with eye symptoms and no abnormality can be found after examination, then he or she must look again as it is likely that something has been missed.

Most of the work of the ophthalmologist is necessarily centred on the globe of the eye itself and there are a number of diseases, which are limited to this region, sometimes without there being any apparent involvement of the rest of the body. Ophthalmology is usually classified as a surgical specialty but it provides a bridge between surgery and medicine. Most of the surgery is performed under the microscope and there is overlap with the fields of the plastic surgeons and the neurosurgeons. On the medical side, the ophthalmologist has links with general physicians, especially when concerned with vascular problems in the eye and diabetes.

Historical Background

In 1847 the English mathematician and inventor, Charles Babbage, showed a distinguished ophthalmologist his device for examining the inside of the eye, but unfortunately this was never exploited and it was not until 1851 that Hermann von Helmholtz published his classic description of his instrument. He developed the idea from his knowledge of optics and the fact that he had previously demonstrated the "red reflex" to medical students with a not dissimilar instrument. It took him about a week to learn the technique of examining in detail the structures within the eye and he wrote a letter to his father at the time telling him that he had made a discovery that was "of the utmost importance to ophthalmology". Soon after this a mass of descriptive information on the optic fundus appeared in the scientific literature and modern clinical ophthalmology was born. The changes in the eye seen in association with systemic diseases such as hypertension and anaemia became recognised. Several blinding conditions limited to the eyes themselves such as glaucoma and macular degeneration were also described at this time.

But we must not belittle developments which had occurred before the invention of the ophthalmoscope. In the eighteenth century considerable advances had been made in the technique and instrumentation of cataract surgery, and the science of optics was being developed to enable the better correction of refractive errors in the eye. The development of ophthalmology in the seventeenth century is revealed in the writings of the diarist Samuel Pepys. Although we have no record of his eye condition other than his own, he did consult an oculist at the time and unfortunately received little comfort or effective treatment. His failing eyesight brought his diary to an abrupt end in spite of the use of "special glasses" and the medicaments, which caused him great pain.

Although records of eye surgical techniques go back as far as 3000 years, modern eye surgery was largely developed thanks to the introduction of cocaine and then of general anaesthesia at the end of the nineteenth century. The use of eserine eyedrops to reduce the intraocular pressure in glaucoma was introduced at the same time, this being the forerunner of a number of different medical treatments, which are now available. Cataract surgery saw great advances at the beginning of the twentieth century with the introduction of the intracapsular cataract extraction. In the 1920s, successful attempts were being made to replace the detached retina, which had previously been an irreversible cause of blindness. Such early surgical techniques have now been developed to produce some of the most dramatic means of restoring sight. As a spin-off from the second world war came a revolutionary idea of "spare parts" surgery in the eye. The observation that injured fighter pilots were able to tolerate small pieces of Perspex in their eyes led to the use of acrylic intraocular implants, the lens of the eye being replaced by an artificial one. Such spare-part surgery has now become commonplace as will be discussed in Chapter 11. The operating microscope was introduced in the 1960s, and with it came the development of fine suture materials and the use of instruments too small for manipulation with the naked eye. Thirty years ago the vitreous was a surgical no-man's land, but instruments have now been developed that can cut, aspirate and inject fluid simultaneously, all these procedures being carried out through fine-bore needles. Membranes, blood or foreign bodies can now be removed from the vitreous as a routine. Much important eye disease is inherited and it is not surprising that very important advances have occurred recently in the field of ophthalmic genetics. The gene controlling the development of the eye has now been identified and perhaps the answer to the tragic problem of inherited degenerative retinal disease is on the horizon.

In the early days of the development of the speciality a number of specialised hospitals were built throughout the UK. The first of these was Moorfield's Eye Hospital, founded largely to combat the epidemic of trachoma, which was prevalent in London at the time. Subsequently other eye hospitals appeared in the main cities, often the result of pressures of local needs such as, for example, the treatment of industrial accidents. In recent years, there has been a tendency for eye departments to become incorporated within the larger district general hospital although individual eye hospitals remain and are still being built.

Basic Anatomy and Physiology of the Eye

2

Introduction

The eye is the primary organ of vision. Each one of the two eyeballs is located in the orbit where it takes up about one-fifth of the orbital volume (Figure 2.1). The remaining space is taken up by the extraocular muscles, fascia, fat, blood vessels, nerves and the lacrimal gland.

The eye is embryologically an extension of the central nervous system. It shares many common anatomical and physiological properties with the brain. Both are protected by bony walls, have firm fibrous coverings and a dual blood supply to the essential nervous layer in the retina. The eye and brain have internal cavities perfused by fluids of similar composition and under equivalent pressures. As the retina and optic nerve are outgrowths from the brain it is not surprising that similar disease processes affect the eye and central nervous system. Physician should constantly remind themselves of the many disease conditions that can simultaneously involve the eye and the central nervous system.

Basic Structure of the Eye and Supporting Structures

The Globe

The eye has three layers or coats, three compartments and contains three fluids (Figure 2.2).

The Three Coats of the Eye

1. Outer fibrous layer
   - cornea
   - sclera
   - lamina cribrosa.
2. Middle vascular layer ("uveal tract")
   - iris
   - ciliary body – consisting of the pars plicata and pars plana
   - choroid.
3. Inner nervous layer
   - pigment epithelium of the retina
   - retinal photoreceptors
   - retinal neurones.

The Three Compartments of the Eye

1. Anterior chamber – the space between the cornea and the iris diaphragm.

2. Posterior chamber – the triangular space between the iris anteriorly, the lens and zonule posteriorly, and the ciliary body laterally.

3. Vitreous chamber – the space behind the lens and zonule.

The Three Intraocular Fluids

1. Aqueous humour – a watery, optically clear solution of water and electrolytes similar to tissue fluids except that aqueous humour typically has a very low protein content.

2. Vitreous humour – a transparent gel consisting of a three-dimensional network of collagen fibres with the interspaces filled with polymerised hyaluronic acid molecules and water. It fills the space between

the posterior surface of the lens, ciliary body and retina.

3. Blood – in addition to its usual functions, blood contributes to the maintenance of intraocular pressure. Most of the blood is in the choroid. The choroidal blood flow represents the largest blood flow per unit tissue in the body. The degree of desaturation of efferent choroidal blood is relatively small and indicates that the choroidal vasculature has functions beyond retinal nutrition. It may be that the choroid serves as a heat exchanger for the retina which absorbs energy as light strikes the retinal pigment epithelium.

Clinically, the Eye may be Considered to be Composed of Two Segments

1. Anterior segment – all structures from (and including) the lens forward.
2. Posterior segment – all structures posterior to the lens.

The Outer Layer of the Eye

The anterior one-sixth of the fibrous layer of the eye is formed by the cornea. The posterior five-sixths is formed by the sclera and lamina cribrosa. The cornea is transparent whereas the sclera, which is continuous within it, is white. The junction of cornea and sclera is known as the limbus. The cornea has five layers anteroposteriorly (Figure 2.3):

1. Epithelium and its basement membrane – stratified squamous type of epithelium with five to six cell layers of regular arrangement.
2. Bowman's layer – homogeneous sheet of modified stroma.
3. Stroma – composes approximately 90% of the total corneal thickness. Consists of lamellae of collagen, cells, and ground substance.
4. Descemet's membrane – the basement membrane of the endothelium.
5. Endothelium – a single layer of cells lining the inner surface of Descemet's membrane.

In the region of the limbus, the epithelium on the outer surface of the cornea becomes continuous with the conjunctiva, a thin, loose transparent mucous membrane which covers the anterior part of the sclera, from which it is separated by loose connective tissue. Above and below, the conjunctiva is reflected on the inner surface of the upper and lower lids. This mucous membrane therefore lines the pos-

terior surface of the eyelids and there is a muco-cutaneous junction on the lid margin. Although the conjunctiva is continuous, it can be divided into three parts: palpebral (tarsal), bulbar and fornix.

The sclera consists of irregular lamellae of collagen fibres. Posteriorly, the external two-thirds of the sclera becomes continuous with the dural sheath of the optic nerve, whilst the inner third becomes the lamina cribrosa – the fenestrated layer of dense collagen fibres through which the nerve fibres pass from the retina to the optic nerve. The sclera is thickest posteriorly and thinnest beneath the insertions of the recti muscles (see Figures 2.1 and 2.2).

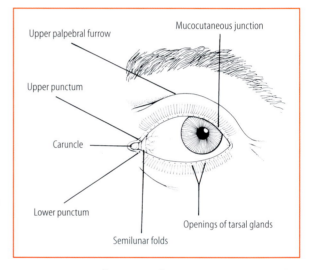

Fig. 2.1.   Surface anatomy.

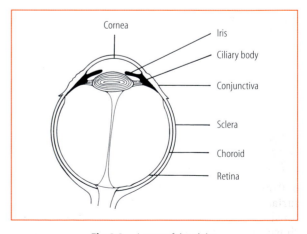

Fig. 2.2.   Layers of the globe.

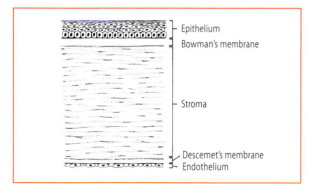

Fig. 2.3.   The cornea.

Middle Layer

The middle layer is highly vascular. If one were to peel the sclera away from this layer (not an easy task), the remaining structure would resemble a grape since this middle layer, which is called the uvea, is heavily pigmented as well as being very vascular. The anterior part of the uvea forms the bulk of the iris body and hence inflammation of the iris is called either anterior uveitis or iritis. The posterior part of the uvea is called the choroid.

The iris is the most anterior part of the uvea. It is a thin, circular disc centrally perforated by the pupil. Contraction of the iris sphincter muscle constricts the pupil while contraction of the dilator pupillae muscle dilates the pupil.

The ciliary body is part of the uveal tissue and is attached anteriorly to the iris and the scleral spur; posteriorly it is continuous with the choroid and retina. The ciliary body is also referred to as the intermediate uvea.

The ciliary body has a triangular cross-section. The anterior side of the ciliary body is the shortest and borders the anterior chamber angle; it gives origin to the iris. The outer side of the triangle (mainly ciliary muscles) lies against the sclera. The inner side is divided into two zones: (1) the pars plicata forms the anterior 2 mm and is covered by ciliary processes and (2) the pars plana constitutes the posterior 4.5 mm flattened portion of the ciliary body. The pars plana is continuous with the choroid and retina.

The choroid consists of:

● Bruch's membrane – membrane on the external surface of the retinal pigment epithelium (RPE). It consists of the basement membrane of RPE cells and choriocapillaris. The elastic and collagenous layers are between the two layers of the basement membrane. Small localised thickenings of Bruch's membrane (which increase with age) are called drusen.
● The choriocapillaris – a network of capillaries supplying the RPE and outer retina.
● Layer of larger choroidal blood vessels external to the choriocapillaris.
● Pigmented cells scattered in the choroid external to the choriocapillaris.

Inner Layer

The inner layer of the eye, which lines the vascular uvea, is the neurosensory layer. This layer forms the retina posteriorly, but anteriorly it comes to line the inner surface of the ciliary body and iris as a two-layered pigment epithelium. These same layers can be traced into the retina, which is composed of an outer pigment epithelium and an inner sensory part which contains the rods and cones, bipolar cells and ganglion cells (Figure 2.4). The junction of the retina and the pars plana forms a scalloped border known as the ora serrata.

It is important to note that the photoreceptor cells are on the outside of the retina. The relationship of the retinal elements can be understood easily by following the formation of the optic cup. As the single-cell layer optic vesicle "invaginates" to form the two-cell layered optic cup, the initially superficial cells become the inner layer of the cup. The pigment epithelium develops from the outer layer of the cup, facing the photoreceptors across the now obliterated

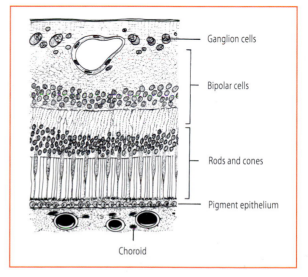

Fig. 2.4.   The retina.

cavity of the optic vesicle. From the inner layer of the optic cup the neurons of the retina differentiate.

Blood Supply

The blood supply of the globe is derived from three sources: the central retinal artery, the anterior ciliary arteries, and the posterior ciliary arteries. All these are derived from the ophthalmic artery which is a branch of the internal carotid. The central retinal artery runs in the optic nerve to reach the interior of the eye and its branches spread over the inner surface of the retina supplying its inner half. The anterior ciliary arteries emerge from the insertion of the recti muscles and perforate the globe near the iris root to join an arterial circle in the ciliary body. The posterior ciliary arteries are the fine branches of the ophthalmic artery, which penetrate the posterior pole of the eye. Some of these supply the choroid and two or more larger vessels run anteriorly to reach the arterial circle in the ciliary body. The larger vessels are known as the long posterior ciliary arteries, and those supplying the choroid are known as the short posterior ciliary arteries. The branches of the central retinal artery are accompanied by an equivalent vein but the choroid, ciliary body and iris are drained by approximately four vortex veins. These leave the posterior four quadrants of the globe and are familiar landmarks for the retina surgeon (Figure 2.5).

Optic Nerve

The optic nerve meets the posterior part of the globe slightly nasal to the posterior pole and very slightly above the horizontal meridian. Inside the eye this point is seen as the optic disc. There are no light-sensitive cells on the optic disc – and hence the blind spot which anyone can find in their field of vision. The optic nerve contains about a million nerve fibres, each of which has a cell body in the ganglion cell layer of the retina (Figure 2.6). Nerve fibres sweep across the innermost part of the retina to reach the optic disc. They can be seen with the ophthalmoscope by carefully observing the way light is reflected off the inner surface of the retina (Figure 2.7). The retinal vessels are also embedded on the inner surface of the retina. There is therefore a gap, which is the thickness of the transparent retina, between the retinal vessels and the stippled pigment epithelium. Apart from the optic nerve, the posterior pole of the globe is also perforated by several long and short ciliary nerves. These contain parasympathetic, sympathetic and sensory fibres, which mainly supply muscles of the iris (dilator and sphincter) and ciliary body (ciliary muscles). Patients can experience pain when the iris is handled under inadequate local anaesthesia, and pain is also sometimes experienced during laser coagulation treatment of the chorioretina – this would seem to prove the existence of sensory fibres in the iris and choroid. The cornea is extremely sensitive, but again, the only sensory endings are those for pain.

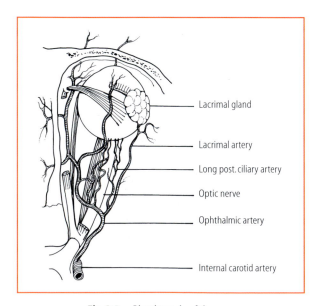

Fig. 2.5.   Blood supply of the eye.

Lacrimal gland

Lacrimal artery

Long post. ciliary artery

Optic nerve

Ophthalmic artery

Internal carotid artery

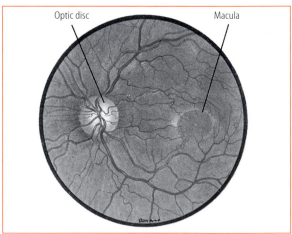

Optic disc

Macula

Fig. 2.6.   The optic fundus.

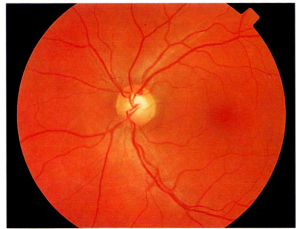

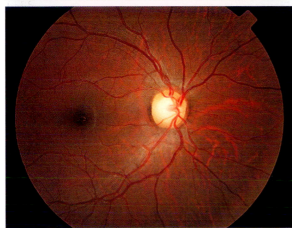

Fig. 2.7. The normal fundus of **a** a Caucasian and **b** an African. The background is darker in the African due to increased pigment in the retinal pigment epithelium. The nerve fibre layer is noticeable especially along the superior and inferior temporal arcades.

The visual pathways include the following.

1. The retina:
   - rods and cones
   - bipolar cells
   - ganglion cells.
2. Axons of the ganglion cells visual and pupillary reflex pathways:
   - nerve fibre layer of retina
   - optic nerve
   - optic chiasm
   - optic tract.
3. Subcortical centres and relays:
   - superior colliculus – reflex control of eye movements

- pretectal nuclei – pupillary reflexes
- lateral geniculate body – cortical relay.

4. Cortical connections
   - optic radiations
   - visual cortex (area 17) – vision and reflex eye movements
   - association areas (areas 18 and 19)
   - frontal eye field – voluntary eye movements.

If the rods and cones are considered analogous to the sensory organs for touch, pressure, temperature, etc. then the bipolar cells may be compared to the first-order sensory neurons of the dorsal root ganglia. By the same token, the retinal ganglion cells can be compared to the second-order sensory neurons, whose cell bodies lie within the spinal cord or medulla.

The Eyelids

The eyelids may be divided into anterior and posterior parts by the mucocutaneous junction – the grey line (Figure 2.8). The eyelashes arise from hair

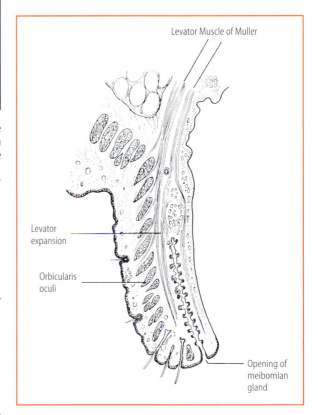

Fig. 2.8. The eyelid.

follicles anterior to the grey line whilst the ducts of the meibomian glands (modified sebaceous glands) open behind the grey line. The meibomian glands are long and slender, and run parallel to each other perpendicular to the eyelid margin and are located in the tarsal plate of the eyelids. The tarsal plate gives stiffness to the eyelids and helps maintain its contour. The upper and lower tarsal plates are about 1 mm thick. The lower tarsus measures about 5 mm in height whilst the upper tarsus measures about 10–12 mm.

The orbicularis oculi muscle lies between the skin and the tarsus and serves to close the eyelids. It is supplied by the facial nerve. The skin and subcutaneous tissue of the lids is very thin. The inner surface of the eyelids is lined by the palpebral conjunctiva.

The Lacrimal Apparatus

The major lacrimal gland occupies the superior temporal anterior portion of the orbit. It has ducts that open into the palpebral conjunctiva above the upper border of the upper tarsus.

Tears collect at the medial part of the palpebral fissure and pass through the puncta and the canaliculi into the lacrimal sac, which terminates in the nasolacrimal duct inferiorly. The nasolacrimal duct opens into the inferior meatus of the nose.

The Extraocular Muscles

There are six extraocular muscles which help to move the eyeball in different directions: the superior, inferior, medial and lateral recti, the superior and inferior obliques. All these muscles are supplied by the IIIrd cranial nerve except the lateral rectus (supplied by the VIth nerve) and superior oblique (IVth nerve).

All the extraocular muscles except the inferior oblique originate from a fibrous ring around the optic nerve (annulus of Zinn) at the orbital apex. The muscles fan out towards the eye to form a "muscle cone". All the recti muscles attach to the eyeball anterior to the equator whilst the oblique muscles attach behind the equator. The optic nerve, the ophthalmic blood vessels and the nerves to the extraocular muscles (except IVth nerve) are contained within the muscle cone (Figure 2.9).

The levator palpebrae superioris is associated with the superior rectus. It arises from just above the annulus of Zinn, runs along the roof of the orbit

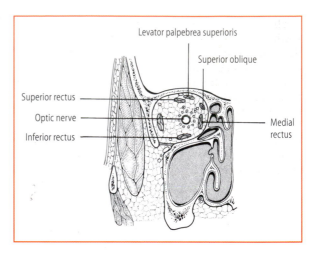

Fig. 2.9.   Anatomy of the orbit.

overlying the superior rectus and attaches to the upper lid skin and anterior surface of the tarsal plate of the upper lid. Tenons capsule is a connective tissue covering which surrounds the eye and is continuous with the fascial covering of the muscles.

Physiology of the Eye

The primary function of the eye is to form a clear image of objects in our environment. These images are transmitted to the brain through the optic nerve and the posterior visual pathways. The various tissues of the eye and its adnexa are thus designed to facilitate this function.

The Eyelids

The functions of the eyelids include: (1) protection of the eye from mechanical trauma, extremes of temperature and bright light and (2) maintenance of the normal precorneal tear film which is important for maintenance of corneal health and clarity.

Normal eyelid closure requires an intact nerve supply to the orbicularis oculi muscles (facial nerve). Eyelid opening is affected by the levator palpebrae superioris supplied by the IIIrd cranial nerve.

The Tear Film

The tear film consists of three layers: the mucoid, aqueous and oily layers.

The mucoid layer lies adjacent to the corneal epithelium. It improves the wetting properties of the tears. It is produced by the goblet cells in the conjunctival epithelium.

The watery (aqueous) layer is produced by the main lacrimal gland in the superotemporal part of the orbit and accessory lacrimal glands found in the conjunctival stroma. This aqueous layer contains electrolytes, proteins, lysozyme, immunoglobulins, glucose and dissolved oxygen (from the atmosphere).

The oily layer (superficial layer of the tear film produced by meibomian glands – modified sebaceous gland) of the eyelid margins. This oily layer helps maintain the vertical column of tears between the upper and lower lids and prevents excessive evaporation.

The tears normally flow away through a drainage system formed by the puncta (inferior and superior), canaliculi (inferior and superior), the common canaliculus, opening into the lacrimal sac, the nasolacrimal duct (which drains into the nose).

The Cornea

The primary function of the cornea is refraction. In order to perform this function, the cornea requires:

1. transparency
2. smooth and regular surface
3. spherical curvature of proper refractive power
4. appropriate index of refraction.

Corneal transparency is contributed to by anatomical and physiological factors.

Anatomical

- Absence of keratinisation of epithelium
- tight packing of epithelial cells
- mucus layer providing smooth lubricated surface
- homogeneity of membranes – Bowman's and Descemet's
- regular arrangement of corneal lamellae (parallel collagen fibres within each lamella with adjacent lamellae being perpendicular)
- regularity produces a diffraction grating
- paucity of corneal stromal cells which are flattened within lamellae
- interspaces: absence of blood vessels.

Physiological

Active dehydration of the cornea through Na^+/HCO_3^- metabolic pump located in the corneal endothelium. This dehydration is supplemented by the physical barrier provided by the corneal epithelium and endothelium.

The Aqueous Humour

The aqueous humour is an optically clear solution of electrolytes (in water) which fills the space between the cornea and the lens. Normal volume is 0.3 ml. Its function is to nourish the lens and cornea.

The aqueous is formed by active secretion and ultrafiltration from the ciliary processes in the posterior chamber. The fluid enters the anterior chamber through the pupil, circulates in the anterior chamber and drains through the trabecular meshwork into the canal of Schlemm, the aqueous veins and the conjunctival episceral veins.

The aqueous normally contains a low concentration of proteins, but a higher concentration of ascorbic acid compared to plasma. Inflammation of the anterior uvea leads to leakage of proteins from the iris circulation into the aqueous (= plasmoid aqueous).

The Vitreous Body

The vitreous consists of a three-dimensional network of collagen fibres with the interspaces filled with polymerised hyaluronic acid molecules which are capable of holding large quantities of water. The vitreous does not normally flow but is percolated slowly by small amounts of aqueous. There is liquefaction of the jelly with age with bits breaking off to form floaters. This degeneration occurs at an earlier age in myopes.

The Lens

The lens, like the cornea, is transparent. It is avascular and depends on the aqueous for nourishment. It has a thick elastic capsule which prevents molecules, for example, proteins moving into or out of it.

The lens continues to grow throughout life – new lens fibres being produced from the outside and moving inwards towards the nucleus with age.

The lens is composed of 65% water and 35% protein. The water content of the lens decreases with age and the lens becomes less pliable.

The lens is suspended from the ciliary body by the zonule which arises from the ciliary body and inserts into the lens capsule near the equator.

The Ciliary Body

The ciliary muscle (within the ciliary body) is a mass of smooth muscle which runs circumferentially inside the globe and is attached to the scleral spur anteriorly. It consists of two main parts: (1) longitudinal (meridional) fibres which form the outer layers and arise from the scleral spur and insert into the choroid. Contraction of this part of the muscle exerts traction on the trabecular meshwork and also the choroid and retina. And (2) circular fibres which form the inner part and run circumferentially.

Contraction moves the ciliary processes inwards towards the centre of the pupil leading to relaxation of the zonules.

Accommodation

Accommodation is the process whereby relaxation of zonular fibres allows the lens to become more globular thereby increasing its refractive power. When the ciliary muscles relax, the zonular fibres become taut and flatten the lens, reducing its refractive power. This is associated with constriction of the pupil and increased depth of focus.

Accommodation is a reflex initiated by visual blurring and/or awareness of proximity of the object of interest. The maximum amount of accommodation (amplitude of accommodation) depends on the rigidity of the lens and contractility of the ciliary muscle. As the lens becomes more rigid with age (and contractions of the ciliary body reduce), accommodation decreases. Reading and other close work become impossible without optical correction – presbyopia.

The Retina

This is the "photographic film" of the eye that converts light into electrical energy (transduction) for transmission to the brain. It consists of two main parts: (1) the neuroretina – all layers of the retina which are derived from the inner layer of the embryological optic cup and (2) the retinal pigment epithelium (RPE) which is derived from the outer layer of the optic cup. It is composed of a single layer of cells which are fixed to Bruch's membrane. Bruch's membrane separates the outer retina from the choroid.

The retinal photoreceptors are located on the outer aspect of the neuroretina, an arrangement which arose from inversion of the optic cup and allows close proximity between the photosensitive portion of the receptor cells and the opaque RPE cells, which reduce light scattering. The RPE also plays an important role in regeneration/recycling of photopigments of the eye and during light–dark adaptation.

In order for the light to reach the photoreceptors to form sharp images, all layers of the retina inner to the photoreceptors must be transparent. This transparency is contributed to by the absence of myelin fibres from the retinal neurones. The axons of the retina ganglion cells normally become myelinated only as they pass through the optic disc to enter the optic nerve.

There are two main types of photoreceptors in the retina: the rods and the cones. In the fovea centralis the only photoreceptors are cones which are responsible for acute vision (visual details) and colour vision. Outside the fovea, rods become more abundant towards the retinal periphery. The rods are responsible for vision in poor (dim) light and for the wide field of vision.

The retinal capillary network (derived from the central retinal artery) extends no deeper than the inner nuclear layer and nourishes the neuroretina from inside up to part of the outer plexiform layer. It is an end-arterial system. The choroid serves to nourish the RPE and the photoreceptors (by diffusion of nutrients). There are no blood vessels in the outer retina. The central fovea is completely avascular and depends on diffusion from the choroidal circulation for its nourishment. Thus normal functioning of the retina requires normal retinal and choroidal circulation.

Examination of the Eye

As in all other medical examinations, examination of a patient with an eye problem should include history, physical examination and special investigation. The age as well as social history, including the patient's occupation should not be forgotten in such an evaluation. A summary of such evaluation is provided in Table 3.1.

How to Find Out What a Patient Can See

One obvious way to measure sight is to ask the patient to identify letters, which are graded in size. This is the basis of the standard Snellen test for visual acuity (Figure 3.1). This test only measures the function of a small area of retina at the posterior pole of the eye called the macula. If we stare fixedly at an object, for example a picture on the wall, and attempt to keep our eyes as still as possible, it soon becomes apparent that we can only appreciate detail in a small part of the centre of the field of vision. Everything around us is ill-defined and yet we can detect the slightest twitch of a finger from the corner of our eyes. The macula region is specialised to detect fine detail, and the whole peripheral retina is concerned with the detection of shape and movement. In order to see, we use the peripheral retina to help us scan the field of view. The peripheral retina may be considered as equivalent to the television cameraman who moves the camera around to the relevant views and allows the camera (or macula) to make sense of the scene. If the macula area is damaged by, for example, senile degeneration, then the patient may be unable to see even the largest print on the test type and yet have

Table 3.1.

History	
Age	
Ophthalmic:	
Subnormal vision	Duration. Difference between eyes.
Disturbances of vision	Distortion, haloes, floaters, flashing lights, momentary losses of vision – field defects.
Pan/discomfort	Increase/decrease
Discharge	Change in appearance – discoloration
Change in Lacrimation	Swelling/mass
	Displacement
Diplopia	
General medical:	Diabetes/hypertension/COAD/dysthyroid/ connective tissue disease
Drugs	FH social/occupational
Examination	
VA: distance/near (with and without glasses)	
Colour vision	
Visual fields	
Orbit	Proptosis/enophthalmos
Ocular movements – conjugate and convergence	Eyelids and lacrimal apparatus
Pupils	Intraocular pressure
Position of eyes	
Conjunctiva, cornea	
AC	
Iris	
Media – lens/vitreous	
Fundus – retina/choroid, optic disc	
Special investigations	
Fluorescein angiography	
Radiological and ultrasound	
Haematological/biochemical/	
Bacteriological/immunological	
Diagnosis	
Anatomic	e.g. cataract
Aetiological	e.g. diabetes

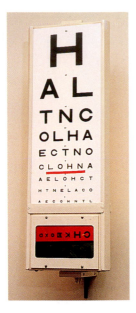

Fig. 3.1.   The Snellen chart.

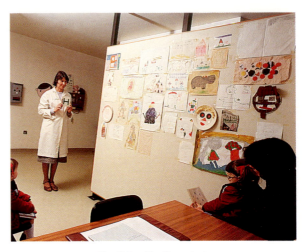

Fig. 3.2.   The Stycar test.

no difficulty in walking about the room. Navigational vision is largely dependent on the peripheral field of vision. On the other side of the coin, the patient with marked constriction of the peripheral field of vision but preservation of the central field may behave as though blind. The same patient could read the test chart down to the bottom *once he has found it*. This situation sometimes arises in patients with advanced chronic simple glaucoma.

It should be becoming clear that measuring the visual acuity alone, although very useful, is not an adequate measure of vision. For a proper clinical examination we need to assess the visual acuity, the visual fields and the colour vision. A number of other facets of visual function can also be measured, such as dark adaptation or the perception of flicker.

Visual Acuity

The familiar Snellen chart has one large letter at the top, which is designed to be just visible to a normal-sighted person at 60 m. The chart is viewed from a distance of 6 m. If a patient is just able to see this large letter, the vision is recorded as 6/60. Below the large letter are rows of smaller letters decreasing in size down to the bottom. The size of letter normally visible to a normal-sighted person at 6 m is usually on the second-to-bottom line. Patients reading this line are said to have a vision of 6/6. If a patient

cannot read the top letter, he is taken nearer to the chart. If the top letter becomes visible at 3 m, the acuity is recorded as 3/60. If the letter is still not visible, the patient is asked if he can count fingers (recorded as "CF") and, failing this, if he can see hand movements ("HM"). Finally, if even hand movements are not seen, the ability to see a light is tested ("P of L").

Young children and illiterates can be asked to do the "E" test in which they must orient a large wooden letter "E" so that it is the same way up as an indicated letter E on a chart. Perhaps better than this is the Stycar test (Figure 3.2) in which the child is asked to point at the letter on a card which is the same as the one held up at 6 m. Other ways of measuring visual acuity are discussed in Chapter 17.

Visual Field

Some measurements of the visual field can be made by sitting facing the patient and asking if the movement of one's fingers can be discerned. The patient is instructed to cover one eye with a hand and the observer also covers one of his eyes so that he can check the patient's field against his own. The test can be made more accurate by using a pin with a red head on it as a target. None of these confrontation methods can match the accuracy of formal perimetry. A number of specialised instruments of varying complexity are available. Using such equipment, the patient is presented with a number of different-sized targets in different parts of the visual field, and a map of the field of vision is charted. An accurate

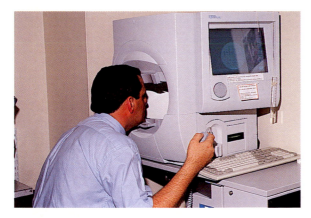

Fig. 3.3. The Humphrey field analyser.

map of the visual field is often of great diagnostic importance. In the past it was customary to map out the central part of the visual field using the Bjerrum screen, and the peripheral field using a perimeter. The Goldmann perimeter was then introduced, and this instrument allows both central and peripheral fields to be plotted out on one chart. The Humphrey field analyser (Figure 3.3) is a further development in field testing. It provides an automated visual field recording system.

Colour Vision

The Ishihara plates provide a popular and effective method for screening for colour vision defects (Figure 3.4). The patient is presented with a series of plates on which are printed numerous coloured dots. The normally sighted subject will see numbers on the majority of the plates, whereas the colour-defective patient will fail to see many of the numbers. The test is easy to do and will effectively screen out the more common red–green deficiency found in 8% of the male population. There are other tests available that will measure blue–green defects, for example, the City University Test. Other tests, such as the Farnsworth 100 Hue test, are available for the more detailed analysis of colour vision.

Spectacles

Measurement of the visual acuity may not be valid unless the patient is wearing the correct spectacles. Some patients when asked to *read* a Snellen chart will put on their reading glasses. Since these glasses are designed for close work, the chart may be largely obscured and the uninitiated doctor might be surprised at the poor level of visual acuity (Figure 3.5). If the glasses have been left at home, long or short sight can be largely overcome by asking the patient to view the chart through a pinhole. Similarly, appropriate spectacle correction (near) must be worn when testing visual fields and colour vision. In an ophthalmic department a check of the spectacle prescription is a routine part of the initial examination. Figure 3.6 shows how the converging power of the optical media and the length of the eye are mismatched to produce the need to wear spectacles.

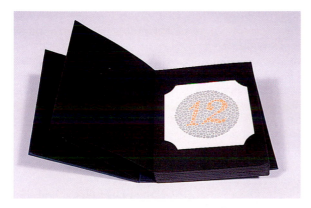

Fig. 3.4. Ishihara plates for colour vision.

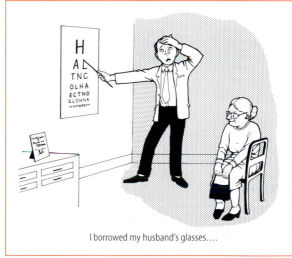

I borrowed my husband's glasses....

Fig. 3.5. The uninitiated may be suprised at the poor level of visual acuity.

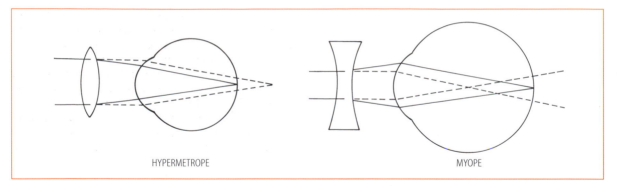

Fig. 3.6. Optical defects of the eye.

How To Start Examining an Eye

Evaluating the Pupil

Examination of the pupil is best performed in a dimly lit room.

Size and symmetry of pupils is assessed by asking the patient to fixate on a distant object such as a letter on the Snellen chart. A dim light is then directed on to the face from below so that both pupils can be seen simultaneously in the diffuse illumination. Normally, the two pupils in any individual are of equal size, although slight differences in size may be observed in up to 20% of the population. Usually physiological unequal pupils (anisocoria) remains unaltered by changing the background illumination.

In order to assess the pupil light reflex a strong focal light is shone on the pupils, one after the other. The direct reaction as well as the consensual reaction (other pupil) are observed. If the afferent arc of the pupil pathway were normal the direct and consensual reactions would be equal.

To assesss the near response of the pupil ask the patient to gaze at a distant object (e.g. Snellen chart) then at a near object (e.g. her own finger-tip just in front of her nose). Observe the pupils as the patient changes gaze from distant to near fixation and vice versa. Generally if the pupil light reflex is intact then the near reflex is normal.

External Eye and Lids

The eyelids should be inspected to make sure that the lid margins and puncta are correctly against the globe and that there are no ingrowing lashes. Rodent ulcers on the skin of the lids can easily be missed, especially if obscured by cosmetics. The presence of ptosis should be noted and the ocular movements assessed by asking the patient to follow a finger upwards, downwards and to each side. Palpation of the skin around the eyes may reveal an orbital tumour or swollen lacrimal sac. Palpation with the end of a glass rod is sometimes useful to find points of tenderness when the lid is diffusely swollen. Such tenderness can indicate a primary infection of a lash root or the lacrimal sac. Both surfaces of the eyelids should be examined. The inside of the lower lid can easily be inspected by pulling down the skin of the lid with the index finger. The upper lid can be everted by asking the patient to look down, grasping the lashes gently between finger and thumb, and rolling the lid margins upwards and forwards over a cotton-wool bud or glass rod. The lid will usually remain in this everted position until the patient is asked to look up. Foreign bodies quite often lodge themselves under the upper lid and they can only be removed by this means. As a general rule, if a patient complains that there is something in her eye, there usually is, and if you find nothing, it is necessary to look again more closely or refer the patient for microscopic examination. A feeling of grittiness may be due to inflammation of the conjunctiva and this may be accompanied by evidence of purulent discharge in the lashes. The presence of tear overflow and excoriation of the skin in the outer canthus should also be noted.

The Globe

Much ophthalmic disease has been described and classified using the microscope. In spite of this, many of the important eye diseases can be diag-

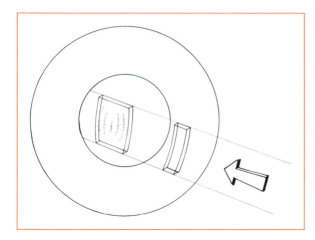

Fig. 3.7. Focal illumination.

nosed using a hand magnifier and an ophthalmoscope. At this point it is important to understand the principle of examining the eye with a focused beam of light. If a pencil of light is directed obliquely through the cornea and anterior chamber, it can be made to illuminate structures or abnormalities otherwise invisible. One might inspect the glass sides and water of a fish tank using a strong, focused torch in the same manner (Figure 3.7). Many ophthalmoscopes incorporate a focused beam of light, which can be used for this purpose. A magnified image of the anterior segment of the eye can be viewed with a direct ophthalmoscope held about 1/3 m away from the eye through a +10 or +12 lens. The principle has been developed to a high degree in the slit-lamp (Figure 3.8). This instrument allows a focused slit of light to be shone through the eye, which can then be examined by a binocular microscope. By this means an optic section of the eye can be created. The method can be compared with making a histological section where the slice of tissue is made with a knife rather than a beam of light. The slit-lamp is sometimes called the biomicroscope. Using such optical aids the cornea must be carefully inspected for scars or foreign bodies. The presence of vascular congestion around the corneal margin may be of significance. Closer inspection of the iris may show that it is atrophic or fixed by adhesions. Turbidity or cells in the aqueous may be seen in the beam of the inspection light. The lens and anterior parts of the vitreous can be examined by the same means.

Once the anterior segment of the eye has been examined, the intraocular pressure is measured. The cheapest way to do this outside an eye department is to use the Schiotz tonometer (Figure 3.9) (for the

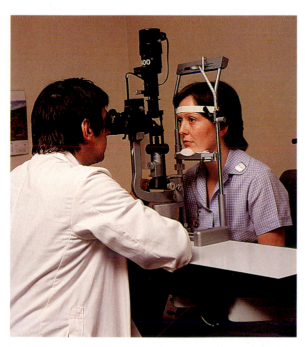

Fig. 3.8. Slit-lamp examination.

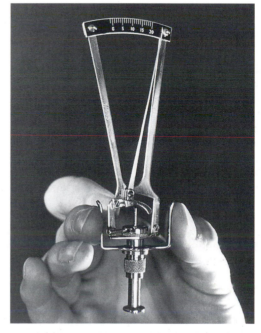

Fig. 3.9. The Schiotz tonometer.

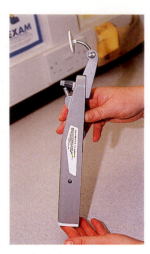

Fig. 3.10. The Perkin's applanation tonometer.

method see Chapter 11). Most optometrists now employ "air-puff" tonometers. This instrument is good for screening but is not as accurate as the applanation tonometer. Applanation tonometry is more accurate and although this instrument is normally attached to the slit-lamp, a hand-held instrument (the Perkins' tonometer) is now available (Figure 3.10).

At this stage, the pupil may be dilated for better examination of the fundi and optical media. A short-acting mydriatic is preferable, for example, tropicamide 1% (Mydriacyl). These particular drops take effect after 10 min and take 2–4 h to wear off. Patients should be warned that their vision will be blurred and that they will be more sensitive to light over this period. Most people find that their ability to drive a car is unimpaired, but there is a potential medicolegal risk if the patient subsequently has a car accident. Once the pupils have been dilated, the eye can then be examined with the ophthalmoscope.

How to Use the Ophthalmoscope

Before the middle of the nineteenth century nobody had seen the inside of a living eye and much of the science of medical ophthalmology was unknown. In 1851 Hermann von Helmholtz introduced his ophthalmoscope and it rapidly became used in clinics dealing with ophthalmological problems. The task of Helmholtz was to devise a way of looking through the black pupil and at the same time illuminate the interior of the globe. He solved the problem by arranging to view the fundus of the eye through an angled piece of glass. A light projected from the side was reflected into the eye by total internal reflection. Most modern ophthalmoscopes employ an angled mirror with a small hole in it to achieve the same end. They also incorporate a series of lenses which can be interposed between the eye of the patient and that of the observer, thereby overcoming any refractive problems which may defocus the view. These lenses are positioned by rotating a knurled wheel at the side of the ophthalmoscope. A number on the face of the instrument indicates the strength of the lens. When choosing an ophthalmoscope, it is worth remembered that large ones take larger batteries which last longer (or, better still, they may have rechargeable batteries); small ophthalmoscopes are handy for the pocket. Some ophthalmoscopes have a wider field of view than others and this is an advantage when learning to use the instrument.

If examining the patient's right eye, it is best to hold the ophthalmoscope in the right hand and view through one's own right eye. A left eye should be viewed with the left eye using the left hand (Figure 3.11). It is best if the patient is seated and the doctor is standing. The first thing to observe is the red reflex, which simply refers to the general reddish colouring seen through the pupil. If viewed from about 30 cm away from the eye, very slight and subtle opacities or defects in the optical media may be seen, against the background of the red reflex. The patient's eye must always be brought into focus by rotating the lens wheel on the ophthalmoscope.

Having observed the red reflex, the eye can be approached closely and the focus of the ophthalmoscope adjusted so that fundus detail becomes visible.

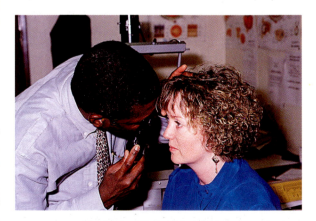

Fig. 3.11. Direct ophthalmoscopy.

It is best to look for the optic disc first, remembering its position nasal to the posterior pole and slightly above the horizontal meridian. The patient should be asked to look straight ahead at this point. The important points to note about the disc are the clarity of the margins, the colour, the nature of the central cup, the vessel entry and the presence or absence of haemorrhages. Once the disc has been examined carefully, the vessels from the disc can be followed. For example, the upper temporal branch vessels can be followed out to the periphery and back, then the lower temporal branch vessels, then the upper nasal and finally the lower nasal. Having examined the vessels, ask the patient to look directly at the ophthalmoscope light and the macular region should some into view. At first this may look unremarkable, like a minute dot of light which follows our own light. More careful examination will reveal that it has a yellowish colour. To obtain a better view of the macular it is usually necessary to examine it with a special attachment on the slip-lamp microscope, the Hruby lens. A fundus photograph is also very helpful. After viewing the macula the general fundus background should be observed. The appearance here depends on the complexion of the patient: in a lightly pigmented subject it is possible to see through the stippled pigment epithelium and obtain an indefinite view of the choroidal vasculature. In heavily pigmented subjects, the pigment epithelium is uniformly black and prevents any view of the choroid, which lies behind it. Finally, the peripheral fundus can be inspected by asking the patient to look to the extremes of gaze and by refocusing the ophthalmoscope. Examining the peripheral fundus demands some special skill, even with the ordinary ophthalmoscope, but it is best seen using the triple mirror gonioscope. This is a modified contact lens which has an angled mirror attached to it. A view through this mirror is obtained using the slit-lamp microscope.

There are a number of other methods of examining the fundus. The ophthalmoscope described above is known as the direct ophthalmoscope. Shortly after the introduction of direct ophthalmoscopy, the indirect ophthalmoscope was introduced. If one examines an eye with the pupil dilated through a mirror with a hole in it, the patient being at arm's length from the observer and the mirror being held close to the observer's eye, then the red reflex is seen. If a convex lens is placed in the line of sight about 8 cm from the patient's eye, then, rather surprisingly, a clear wide field inverted view of the fundus is obtained. The view can be made binocular,

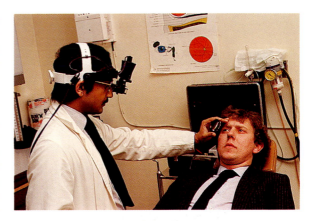

Fig. 3.12. Indirect ophthalmoscopy.

and the binocular indirect ophthalmoscope is an essential tool of the retinal surgeon (Figure 3.12). If we want a really magnified view of the fundus, then the slit-lamp microscope can be used. However, a special lens must be placed in front of the patient's eye, either in the form of the triple mirror contact lens (Figure 3.13) or the Hruby lens. Furthermore, fundus biomicroscopy may also utilise strong convex lenses e.g. VOLK +60, +78 or +90DS aspheric lenses. These high power convex lenses provide inverted reversed images like the indirect ophthalmoscope. Another useful way of examining the fundus is by means of fundus photography. The photographs provide a permanent record of the fundus. A special type of fundus photograph known as a fluorescein angiogram shows up the retinal vessels, including the capillaries, in great detail. The tech-

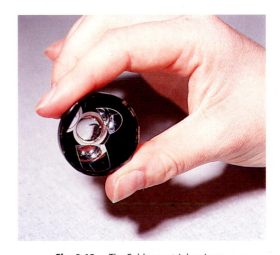

Fig. 3.13. The Goldmann triple mirror.

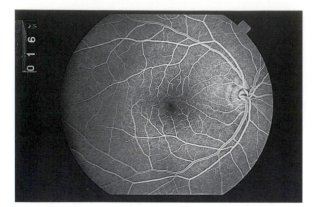

Fig. 3.14. Fluorescein angiogram of normal fundus.

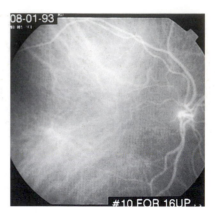

Fig. 3.15. Indocyanine green angiography of normal fundus.

nique involves taking repeated photographs in rapid succession after the injection of the dye fluorescein into the antecubital vein. The dye in the vessels is selectively photographed by using filters in the camera (Figure 3.14). Indocyanine green angiography (ICG) is more useful in assessing the choroidal circulation since ICG-A fluorescence is transmitted through the retinal pigment epithelium (compared to fluorescein) (Figure 3.15). Video filming is becoming an important method for observing changing events in the fundus and it is now possible to view a real time image of the optic fundus on a television screen using the scanning laser ophthalmoscope. This type of equipment will undoubtedly become a routine tool for the ophthalmologist.

Other Tests Available in an Eye Department

Several special tests are available to measure the ability of the eyes to work together. A department known as the orthoptic department is usually set aside within the eye clinic for making these tests. When there is a defect of the ocular movements, this can be monitored by means of the Hess chart (see Chapter 14 on squint). The ability to use the eyes together is measured on the synoptophore, and any tendency of one eye to turn out or in can be measured with the Maddox rod and Maddox wing test (Figure 3.16). The use of contact lenses and also of intraocular implants has demanded more accurate measurements of the cornea and of the length of the eye. A keratometer is an instrument for measuring

the curvature of the cornea, and the length of the eye can now be accurately measured by ultrasound. If one eye appears to protrude forwards and one wishes to monitor the position of the globes relative to the orbital margin, then an exophthalmometer is used (Figure 3.17). X-rays of the eye and orbit are still used. An X-ray is essential if an intraocular foreign body is suspected and it is useful for detecting bony abnormalities in the walls of the orbit due to tumours. Computerised tomography (CT) scanning has become an important diagnostic technique, especially for lesions in the orbit (Figure 3.18) particularly those involving bony tissues. This specialised X-ray has surpassed plain X-rays for most ophthalmic purposes. Magnetic resonance imaging (MRI) is more useful in assessing soft tissues of the orbit and cranium. Ultrasonography is a technique for measuring the length of the eye; it may also be

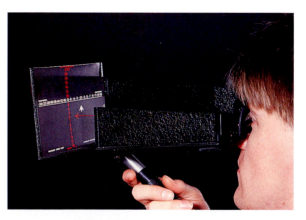

Fig. 3.16. The Maddox wing.

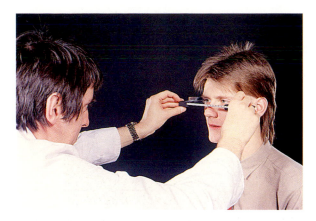

Fig. 3.17. The exophthalmometer.

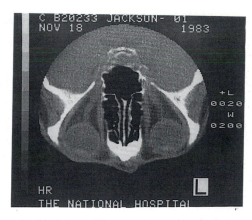

Fig. 3.18. Computerised tomography scan of eyes and orbit (normal).

used to depict tissue planes within the eye, showing for example the extent of a retinal detachment or the presence of vitreous membranes. It can used to determine the presence or absence of retinal diseases especially in eyes with opaque media, for example, cataract or vitreous haemorrhage. It is also useful in characterising tissues of the eye and orbit, for example, choroidal melanomas. Electroretinography provides a measure of the electrical changes which take place in the retina when the eye is exposed to light. It can indicate retinal function in the same way

that the electrocardiogram indicates cardiac function. The visually evoked potential (VEP) is a measure of minute electrical changes over the back of the scalp which occur when the eyes are stimulated with a flashing light. This test has been shown to be useful in detecting previous damage to the optic nerve in patients with suspected multiple sclerosis.

The eye is probably the most measured organ in the body. There are many other ingenious instruments that are not in regular clinical use but which may be found in the laboratory.

Section II

Primary Eye Care Problems

The aim of this section is to present some of the more commonly occurring eye conditions which are likely to confront a casualty officer in the general or eye casualty department, or a general practitioner in his or her surgery. Some of the conditions can also be treated at primary care level, but referral for more extensive investigation and treatment is often required.

Long Sight, Short Sight ⓸

When the patient with an ophthalmological problem first enters the doctor's surgery, it is useful to notice whether he or she is long or short sighted. The long-sighted person tends to have physically smaller eyes than normal with an anteroposterior diameter of less than 24 mm (hypermetropia) whereas the short-sighted person has physically larger eyes than normal with an anteroposterior diameter of more than 24 mm (myopia). Nonetheless the long-sighted

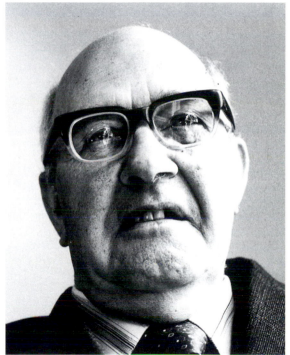

Fig. 4.2. A short-sighted person.

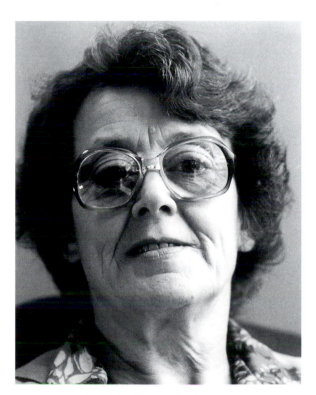

Fig. 4.1. A long-sighted person.

or hypermetropic patient has to wear corrective convex lenses which make the eyes *look* bigger whereas the myopic patient has to wear concave lenses which make the eyes look smaller (Figures 4.1 and 4.2). Glasses, which magnify the eyes, belong to the hypermetrope. The nature of the spectacle correction lens can be verified by moving it backwards and forwards in front of one's hand. If the hand appears to move in the opposite direction to that of the movement of the spectacle lens, it is convex

25

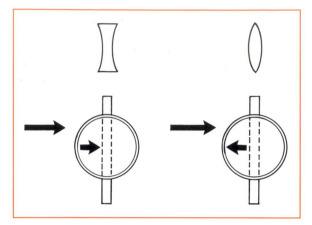

Fig. 4.3. Concava lens "with"; convex lens "against". Try this for yourself in the clinic.

(Figure 4.3). The spectacles of the myopic (or short-sighted) patient contain diverging concave lenses and if these are held in front of one's hand and moved to and fro, the hand appears to move with the direction of the movement of the glasses. After a little practice it is possible to recognise long- or short-sighted patients simply by looking at them, providing that the glasses they are wearing are strong enough (Figure 4.4). This simple observation is helpful in making a diagnosis because myopic and hypermetropic individuals are susceptible to different eye conditions.

Myopia and hypermetropia must not be confused with presbyopia, which is the failure of the eyes to focus on near objects, which comes with increasing

age. It has nothing to do with the length of the eyeball but is related to the diminished ability to change the shape of the lens. Obviously myopes, hypermetropes and those with no refractive error are all susceptible to presbyopia.

The long-sighted person unlike the myope may be predisposed to developing acute narrow angle glaucoma especially in late middle age. The optic disc of the long-sighted person tends to be smaller and pinker and in extreme cases, especially in children, can look swollen when it is not. By contrast the optic disc of the myope is larger and paler with well-defined margins and can be mistaken for an atrophic disc.

Short-sighted patients are more susceptible to retinal detachment, especially in late middle age; they are also more likely to develop cataracts in later years than are people with normal sight.

Table 4.1 gives a list of some of those conditions, which are more commonly associated with either myopia or hypermetropia.

Having observed the nature of the spectacle lenses we have now made a small step towards diagnosing the eye condition. If the patient is middle aged and complaining of evening headaches, seeing haloes around street lights and at the same time blurring of vision then narrow angle glaucoma is the wrong diagnosis if the patient is myopic. If the patient in Figure 4.2 were to be complaining of the sudden appearance of black spots combined with seeing flashes of light he may be about to have a retinal detachment.

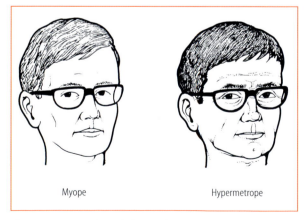

Myope   Hypermetrope

Fig. 4.4. Long sight and short sight. Note the line of the cheek behind the lens.

Table 4.1. Eye disease and refractive error

Myopia ("short sight")	Hypermetropia ("long sight")
Conditions associated with myopia	Conditions associated with hypermetropia
Retinal detachment	Narrow angle glaucoma
Macula haemorrhages	Concomitant squint
Cataract	Amblyopia of disuse
Myopic chorioretinal degeneration	
Down's syndrome	
keratoconus (conical cornea)	
Conditions causing myopia	Conditions causing hypermetropia
Large eye	Small eye
Cataract	Retinal detachment
Diabetes mellitus	Orbital tumours
Accommodation Spasm, or 'pseudomyopia'	Macula oedema
Congenital glaucoma	

If we take note of whether a patient is long or short sighted at an early stage, then this information can influence the type of questions that are best asked when taking a history.

Finally it is worth remembering that the myopic patient can see objects close at hand and read without glasses at any age whereas the hypermetropic patient has to focus to see at all distances. If the hypermetrope has good focusing power (i.e. the younger subject) then the distance vision may be clear without glasses but when hypermetropia is more severe the unaided vision is poor at all ranges.

Common Diseases of the Eyelids 5

The Watering Eye

Quite often patients present at the clinic or surgery complaining of watering eyes. It may be the golfer whose glasses keep misting up on the fairway or the housewife who is embarrassed by tears dropping on food when cooking, or it may be the six-month-old baby whose eyes have watered and discharged since birth. Sometimes an elderly patient may complain of watering eyes when on examination there is no evidence of tear excess but the vision has been made blurred by cataracts. Some degree of tear overflow is of course quite normal in windy weather, and the anxious patient may over-emphasise this; it is important to assess the actual amount of overflow by asking the patient whether it occurs all the time both in and out of doors.

An eye may water because the tears cannot drain away adequately or because there is excessive secretion of tears.

Impaired Drainage of Tears

Normally the tears drain through two minute openings at the inner end of the lid margins known as the upper and lower lacrimal puncta.

The Lacrimal Passageway

Most of the tears drain through the lower punctum. The puncta mark the opening of the lacrimal canaliculi and these small tubes conduct tears medially to the common canaliculus and thence into the tear sac (Figure 5.1). The tear sac is connected directly to the nasolacrimal duct, which opens into the inferior meatus of the nose below the inferior turbinate

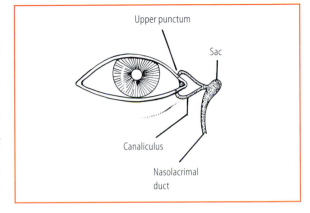

Fig. 5.1.   The lacrimal passageway.

bone. The lacrimal puncta are easily visible to the naked eye and in the elderly the opening of the lower punctum may appear to project upwards like a miniature volcano. Inadequate drainage of tears may be due to displacement of the punctum; the lower lid in the elderly sometimes becomes turned inwards (entropion) due to the fact that the whole tarsal plate rotates on a horizontal axis (Figure 5.2). This in turn is due to slackening of the fascial attachments of the lower margin of the tarsal plate. At first the eyelid turns in whenever the patient screws up the eyes but eventually the lid becomes permanently turned in so that the lashes are no longer visible externally and rub on the cornea. Such patients complain of watering sore eyes and the matter can be corrected very effectively by eyelid surgery. Entropion may also result from scarring and contracture of the conjunctiva on the inner surface of the eyelid.

Not only may the punctum become turned inwards, but it may also be turned outwards. Sometimes the

29

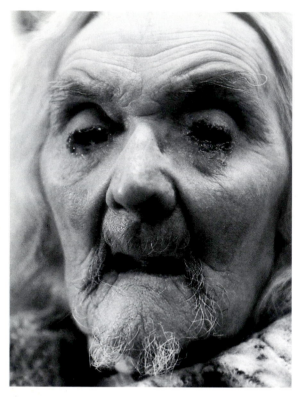

Fig. 5.2. Bilateral entropion. The inturned lower eyelids are largely obscured by purulent discharge.

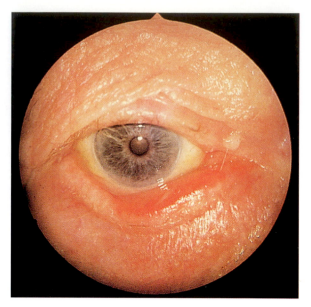

Fig. 5.3. Ectropion.

eversion may be very slight but enough to cause problems. Sometimes the patient may have been using eyedrops, which combined with the overflow of tears causes excoriation and contracture of the skin of the lower eyelid. This leads to further eversion or ectropion of the lower eyelid (Figure 5.3). Often the ectropion arises as the result of increasing laxity of the skin in the elderly but it may also be due to scarring and contracture of the skin due to trauma (cicatricial ectropion). Ectropion may be corrected very effectively by suitable lid surgery.

Drainage of tears along the lacrimal canaliculi depends to some extent on the muscular action of certain fibres of the orbicularis oculi muscle. This band of fibres encloses the lacrimal sac and it is thought that the walls of the sac are thereby stretched, producing slight suction along the canaliculi. Whatever the exact mechanism, when the orbicularis muscle is paralysed the tear flow is impaired even if the position of the punctum is normal. Sometimes patients who have suffered a Bell's palsy may complain of a watering eye even though they appear to have otherwise made a complete recovery.

Misplacement of the drainage channels, particularly of the punctum, may thus affect the outflow of tears, but perhaps more commonly the drainage channel itself becomes blocked. In young infants with lacrimal obstruction the blockage is usually at the lower end of the nasolacrimal duct and takes the form of a plug of mucus or a residual embryological septum which has failed to become naturally perforated. In these cases there is nearly always some purulent discharge which may be expressed from the tear sac by gentle pressure with the index finger over the medial palpebral ligament. The mother is shown how to express this material once or twice daily and is instructed to instil antibiotic drops three or four times daily. This treatment alone may resolve the problem and many cases may undoubtedly resolve spontaneously. Sometimes it is necessary to syringe and probe the tear duct under a short anaesthetic. Usually one waits until the child is at least six months old before considering probing. In adults the obstruction is more often in the common canaliculus or nasolacrimal duct. In these cases the tear duct can be syringed after the instillation of local anaesthetic drops. This procedure is simple though it must be done with care to avoid damaging the canaliculus, and even if the obstruction is not cleared it can allow the surgeon to identify the site of

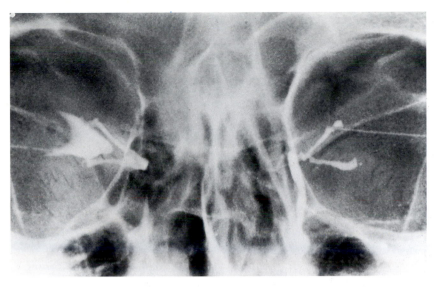

Fig. 5.4.   Dacryocystogram (with acknowledgement to Mr R. Welham).

the obstruction. Sometimes a permanent obstruction is identified at the lower end of the naso-lacrimal duct, which can be relieved by surgery under general anaesthesia or the more recently introduced laser treatment applied through the nose. The initial investigation of lacrimal obstruction entails syringing and if this does not give the information required, it is possible to display the tear duct by X-ray using a radio-opaque contrast medium. This is injected into the lower canaliculus with a lacrimal syringe (Figure 5.4). The technique is known as dacryocystography.

Acute Dacryocystitis

Sometimes the lacrimal sac may become infected. This may occur in either children or adults but is more common in adult females. The condition may present initially as a watering eye and, in its early stages, the diagnosis may be missed if the tear sac is not gently palpated and found to be tender. Subsequently there is marked swelling and tenderness at the inner canthus and eventually the abscess may point and burst. In its early stages the condition can be aborted by the use of local and systemic antibiotics, but once an abscess has formed this may point and burst on the skin surface. Surgical incision and drainage of a lacrimal abscess can lead to the formation of a lacrimal fistula (Figure 5.5).

Very rarely, the lacrimal canaliculi may become infected by the fungus Actinomycosis and a small

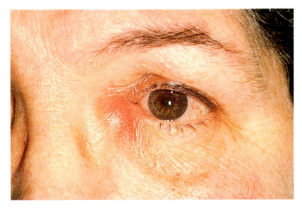

Fig. 5.5.   Acute dacryocystitis (with acknowledgement to Mr R. Welham).

tell-tale bead of pus can be expressed from the punctum. The condition is very resistant to ordinary treatment with local antibiotics, and is best treated by opening up the punctum with a fine knife especially designed for the purpose – the procedure being called canaliculotomy – and then irrigating the canaliculi and tear duct with a suitable antibiotic.

The diagnosis of lacrimal obstruction therefore depends first on an examination of the eyelids, secondly on syringing the tear ducts, and then if necessary dacryocystography. Figure 5.6 illustrates the diagnostic use of lacrimal syringing.

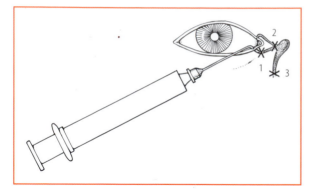

Fig. 5.6. Diagnostic use of lacrimal syringing. (1) Obstruction in canaliculus shown by regurgitation of saline back through punctum. (2) Common canaliculus obstruction shown by return of saline through upper punctum. (3) Obstruction in nasolacrimal duct shown by filling of lacrimal sac.

Excessive Secretion of Tears

A wide range of conditions affecting the eye may cause an excessive production of tears, from acute glaucoma to a corneal abscess, but these do not usually present as a watering eye since the other symptoms such as pain or visual loss are more evident to the patient. Occasionally the unwary doctor may be caught out by an irritative lesion on the cornea, which mimics the more commonplace lacrimal obstruction. For example, a small corneal foreign body or an ingrowing eyelash may present in this way. Not uncommonly, a loose lash may float into the lower lacrimal canaliculus where it may become lodged causing chronic irritation at the inner canthus. Its removal after weeks of discomfort produces instant relief and gratitude.

The Dry Eye

A patient may complain of dryness of the eyes simply because the conjunctiva is inflamed, but when the tear film really is defective the patient may complain of soreness and irritation rather than dryness. The diagnosis of a dry eye depends on a careful examination and it is quite erroneous to assume that the tear film is inadequate simply because the patient complains of dryness, or even if the symptoms appear to be improved by artificial tears.

The normal tear film is in three layers and the integrity of this film is essential for comfort and more important for good vision. The anterior or outermost layer is formed by the oily secretion of the meibomian glands and the layer next to the cornea is mucinous to allow proper wetting by the watery component of the tears which lies sandwiched between the two. This three-layered film is constantly maintained by the act of blinking.

Causes

- Systemic disease with lacrimal gland involvement.
  - sarcoidosis
  - rheumatoid arthritis (Sjögren's syndrome).
- Trachoma (chlamydial conjunctivitis and keratitis – see the next chapter).
- Neuroparalytic keratitis.
- Exposure keratitis.
- Old age.
- Other rare causes.

Signs

Slit-lamp Examination

In a normal subject the tear film is evident as a rim of fluid along the lid margin and a deficiency of this may be seen by direct examination. Prolonged deficiency of tears may be associated with the presence of filaments – microscopic strands of mucus and epithelial cells, which stain with Rose Bengal. Punctate staining of the corneal epithelium is also seen after applying a drop of fluorescein. In some dry eye syndromes, for example, ocular pemphigoid and Stevens–Johnson syndrome, keratinisation of the cornea and conjunctiva with the formation of contracting adhesions between the opposed surfaces of the conjunctiva occurs. A similar change is apparent following chemical or thermal burns of the eyes.

Schirmer's Test

One end of a special filter paper strip is placed between the globe and the lower eyelid. The other end projects forward and the time taken for the tears to wet the projecting strip is measured. The test is not a very accurate measure of tear secretion but it provides a useful guide (Figure 5.7).

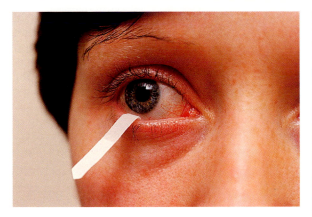

Fig. 5.7. Schirmer's test.

Tear Film Break-up Time

Using the slit-lamp microscope, the time for the tear film to break up when the patient stops blinking is measured. This test is sometimes used as an index of mucin deficiency.

Management of the Dry Eye

This, of course, depends on the cause of the dry eye and the underlying systemic cause may require treatment in the first place. Artificial tear drops are a mainstay in treatment and various types are available, their use depending on which component of the tear film is defective. In severe cases it may be necessary to consider temporary or permanent occlusion of the lacrimal puncta

Deformities of the Eyelids

The Normal Eyelid

Figure 5.8 is a diagram of the normal eyelid in cross-section. The lids contain two antagonistic voluntary muscles; the more superficial orbicularis oculi, supplied by the seventh cranial nerve, which closes the eye, and the tendon of the levator palpebrae superioris supplied by the third cranial nerve, which opens the eye. We must not forget that there is also some smooth muscle in the upper and lower eyelids, which has clinical importance apart from its influence on facial expression when the subject is under stress. Loss of tone in this muscle accounts for the slight ptosis seen in Horner's syndrome; increased

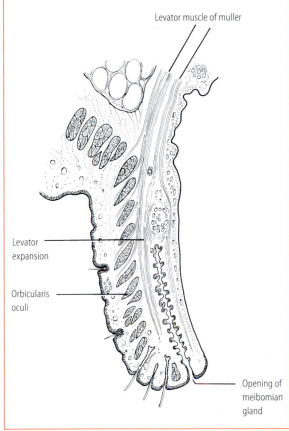

Fig. 5.8. Cross-section of a normal eyelid.

tone is seen in thyrotoxic eye disease. These muscles (that in the upper lid is known as Müller's muscle) are attached to the skeleton of the lid which is the tarsal plate, a plate of fibrous tissue (not cartilage) which contains the meibomian glands.

Epicanthus

Figure 5.9 shows that this is characterised by vertical folds of skin at the inner canthus. These folds are seen quite commonly in otherwise quite normal infants and they gradually disappear as the facial bones develop. Children with epicanthus may appear to the uninitiated to be squinting and this can cause considerable parental anxiety. It is important to explain that the squint is simply an optical illusion once the absence of any true deviation of the eyes has been confirmed. Epicanthus persists into adult life in Mongolian races, and occasionally it is seen in

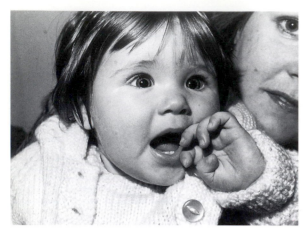

Fig. 5.9. Epicanthus

European adults. It may also be associated with other eyelid deformities.

Entropion

This is an inturning of the eyelid. The common form is the inturning of the lower eyelid seen in elderly patients. Often the patient does not notice that the eyelid is inturned but complains of soreness and irritation. Closer inspection reveals the inturned eyelid, which can be restored to its normal position by slight downward pressure on the lower eyelid, only to turn in again when the patient forcibly closes the eyes. The inturned eyelashes tend to rub on the cornea and if neglected the condition can lead to corneal scarring and consequent loss of vision. The condition is often associated with muscular eyelids and sometimes seems to be precipitated by repeatedly screwing up the eyes. Slackening of the fascial sling of the lower eyelid with ageing combined with the action of the orbicularis muscle allows this to happen. This common type of entropion is called spastic entropion and it can be promptly cured without leaving a visible scar by minor eyelid surgery. Entropion may also be seen following scarring of the conjunctival surface of the eyelids and one must mention in particular the entropion of the upper eyelid caused by trachoma. This is very rare in the UK but still common in the Middle East and countries where trachoma is still rife.

Ectropion

This commonly seen outward turning of the lower eyelid in the elderly is eminently treatable and responds well to minor surgery. Senile ectropion may begin with slight separation of the lower eyelid from the globe, and the malposition of the punctum leads to overflow of tears and conjunctival infection. Irritation of the skin by the tears and rubbing of the eyes leads to skin contracture and further downward pulling of the eyelids. Like entropion, ectropion may be cicatricial and result from scarring of the skin of the eyelids. It may also follow a seventh cranial nerve palsy due to complete inaction of the orbicularis muscle; this is called paralytic ectropion.

Lagophthalmos

This is the term used to denote failure of proper closure of the eyelids due to inadequate blinking or lid deformity. In all these cases the cornea is inadequately lubricated and exposure keratitis may develop. If untreated this can lead to a serious situation; initially the cornea shows punctate staining when a drop of fluorescein is placed in the conjunctival sac and subsequently a corneal ulcer may appear. This in turn can lead to the spread of infection into the eye and without prompt treatment with antibiotics the eye may eventually be lost.

As a general principle it is important to realise that the sight may be lost simply because the eyes cannot blink. The principle applies especially to the unconscious or the anaesthetised patient where a disaster may be avoided by taping or padding the eyelids and applying an antibiotic ointment.

Blepharospasm

Slight involuntary twitching of the eyelids is very common and not usually considered to be of any pathological significance other than being a symptom of fatigue or sometimes of an anxiety state. The condition is termed "myokymia". True blepharospasm is rare. It may be unilateral or bilateral and may cause great inconvenience and worry to the patient. It tends slowly to become more marked over many years. A small proportion of patients eventually develops Parkinsonism. Cases of recent onset need to be investigated because they may be due to an intracranial space-taking lesion. In most cases though no underlying cause can be found. Patients with this type of blepharospasm (essential blepharospasm) can often be treated quite effectively by injecting small doses of botulinum toxin into the eyelids, but these need to be repeated every few months.

Redundant Lid Skin

Excessive skin on the eyelids is commonly seen in elderly people, often as a family characteristic. It may result from chronic oedema of the eyelids due, for example, to thyrotoxic eye disease or to renal disease. The problem is made worse in some cases by herniation of orbital fat through the orbital septum, and excision of the redundant skin and orbital fat may sometimes be necessary.

Ptosis

Drooping of one upper lid is an important clinical sign. In ophthalmic practice, ptosis in children is usually congenital and in adults is either congenital or due to a third cranial nerve palsy. These more common causes must always be kept in mind but there are a large number of other possible ones. When confronted with a patient whose upper lid appears to droop the first thing to decide is whether the eyelid really is drooping or whether the lid on the other side is retracted. The upper lid may droop because the eye is small and hypermetropic or shrunken from disease. Having eliminated the possibility of such "pseudoptosis", the various other causes can be considered beginning on the skin of the eyelid – styes, meibomian cysts – and advancing centrally through muscle – myasthenia gravis – along nerves – oculomotor palsy, Horner's syndrome – to the brainstem. Marked ptosis with the eye turned down and out and a dilated pupil is an oculomotor palsy whereas very slight ptosis, often not noticed by the patient or sometimes by the doctor, is more likely to mean Horner's syndrome. This syndrome is due to damage to the sympathetic nervous supply to either upper or lower lids or both and is characterised by slight ptosis, small pupil, loss of sweating on the affected side of the face and slight enophthalmos (posterior displacement of the globe).

The management of ptosis depends on the cause and thus on accurate diagnosis. Surgical shortening of the levator tendon is effective in some cases of congenital ptosis and sometimes in long-standing third cranial nerve palsies. Before embarking on surgery it is important to exclude myasthenia gravis and corneal anaesthesia. Children with congenital ptosis need to be assessed very carefully before considering surgery. In young children ptosis surgery is indicated where the drooping lid threatens to cover the line of sight and where the ptosis causes an unacceptable backwards tilt of the head. In one rather strange type of congenital ptosis, the problem disappears when the mouth is opened and the patient may literally wink unavoidably when chewing. Careful consideration is needed before making the decision for surgery in these cases.

Causes of Ptosis

- Pseudoptosis: small eye, atrophic eye, lid retraction on other side.
- Mechanical ptosis: inflammation, tumour, and excess skin.
- Myogenic ptosis: myasthenia gravis.
- Neurogenic ptosis: sympathetic – Horner's syndrome, IIIrd cranial nerve palsy, any lesion in the pathway of these, carcinoma of the lung may cause Horner's syndrome.
- Drugs: guanethidine eye drops cause ptosis.
- Congenital: ask for childhood photograph, ask for family history.

Ingrowing Eyelashes (Trichiasis)

The lashes may grow in an aberrant manner even though the eyelids themselves are in good position. This may be the result of chronic infection of the lid margins or may follow trauma. Sometimes one or two aberrant lashes appear for no apparent reason (Figure 5.10). The lashes tend to rub on the cornea

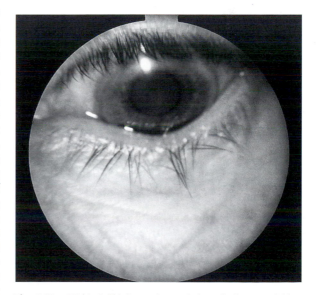

Fig. 5.10.   Trichiasis. This ingrowing eyelash on the lower eyelid has been causing a sore eye for three months.

producing irritation and secondary infection. The condition is referred to as "trichiasis". When one or two lashes are found to be the cause of the patients discomfort, it is common practice simply to epilate them with epilating forceps. This produces instant relief, but often the relief is short-lived because the lashes regrow. At this stage the best treatment is to destroy the lash roots by electrolysis prior to epilation. Needless to say, before removing lashes it is essential to be familiar with the normal position of the lash line and to realise, for example, that hairs are normally present on the caruncle! When the lash line is grossly distorted by injury or disease, the rubbing of the lashes on the cornea can be prevented by fitting a protective contact lens or, if this measure proves impractical, it may be necessary to transpose or excise the lashes and their roots.

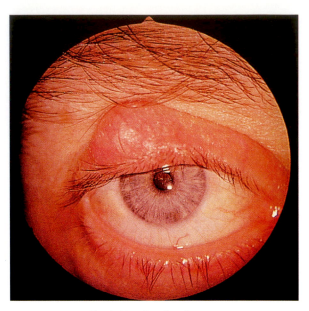

Fig. 5.11. A meibomian cyst.

Infections of the Eyelids

Meibomian Gland Infection

The opening of the meibomian glands may become infected at any age resulting in meibomitis, seen initially as redness along the line of a gland when the eyelid is everted. A small abscess may then form with swelling and redness of the whole eyelid and this may point and burst either through the conjunctiva or less often through the skin. The orifice of a gland may become occluded and the gland then becomes distended and cystic. The retained secretions of the gland set up a granulating reaction and the cyst itself may become infected. The patient may complain of soreness and swelling of the eyelid which subsides leaving a pea-sized swelling which remains for many months and sometimes swells up again. During the stage of acute infection the best treatment is local heat preferably in the form of steam. This produces considerable relief and is preferable to the use of systemic or local antibiotics. Antibiotics may be required if the patient has several recurrences or if there are signs and symptoms of septicaemia. Once a pea-sized cyst remains in the tarsal plate, this can be promptly removed under a local anaesthetic unless the patient is a child in which case a general anaesthetic may be required. The method of removal involves everting the eyelid and incising the cyst through the conjunctiva and then curetting the contents. Postoperatively, local antibiotic drops or ointment are prescribed (Figure 5.11).

Styes

These are distinct from meibomian infections, being the result of infection of the lash root. The eyelid may swell up and become painful and at this stage the site of the infection may be uncertain. However, a small yellow pointing area is eventually seen around the base of an eyelash. Hot steaming again is effective treatment and once the pus is seen the eyelash can be gently epilated with resulting discharge and subsequent resolution of the infection.

Children aged from about 6–10 years sometimes seem to go through periods of their lives when they may be dogged by recurrent styes and meibomian infections, much to the distress of the parents. Under these conditions very frequent baths and hair-washing are advised and sometimes a long-term systemic antibiotic may be considered. Recurrent lid infections may raise the suspicion of diabetes mellitus but in practice this is rarely found to be an underlying cause.

Eyelid infections such as these very rarely cause any serious problems other than a day or two off work and it is extremely unusual for the infection to spread and cause orbital cellulitis. Recurrent swelling of the eyelid in spite of treatment may indicate the need for a lid biopsy because some malignant tumours may on rare occasions present in a deceptive manner.

Blepharitis

This refers to a chronic inflammation of the lid margins due to staphylococcal infection. The eyes become red rimmed and there is usually an accumulation of scales giving the appearance of fine dandruff on the lid margins. The condition is often associated with seborrhoea of the scalp. Sometimes it becomes complicated by recurrent styes or chronic infection of the meibomian glands. The eye itself is not usually involved although there may be a mild superficial punctate keratitis as evidenced by fine staining of the lower part of the cornea with fluorescein. In more sensitive patients the unsightly appearance may cause difficulties, but in more severe cases the discomfort and irritation may interfere with work. Severe recurrent infection may lead to irregular growth of the lashes and trichiasis.

In the management of these patients it is important to explain the chronic nature of the condition and the fact that certain individuals seem to be prone to it. Attention should be given to keeping the hair, face and hands as clean as possible and to avoid rubbing the eyes. When the scales are copious they can be gently removed with cotton-wool moistened in sodium bicarbonate lotion twice daily. Dandruff of the scalp should also be treated with a suitable shampoo. A local antibiotic may be applied to the lid margins twice daily with good effect in many but not all cases. In severe cases with ulceration of the lid margin it may be necessary to consider prescribing a systemic antibiotic preferably after identifying the causative organism by taking a swab from the eyelids. Local steroids when combined with a local antibiotic are very effective treatment, but the prescriber must be aware of the dangers of using steroids on the eye and long-term treatment with steroids should be avoided. Steroids should not be used without monitoring the intraocular pressure.

Molluscum Contagiosum

This is a viral infection usually seen in children. The lesions on the eyelids are discrete, slightly raised and umbilicated and usually multiple. There are also likely to be lesions elsewhere on the body, especially the hands; and siblings may have the same problem. It is rare for the eye itself to be involved. The best treatment for a child is the curettage of each lesion under a general anaesthetic.

Orbital Cellulitis

Although this is not strictly a lid infection it may be confused with severe meibomitis. The infection is deeper and the implications much more serious. In a child where the condition is more common, there is eyelid swelling, pyrexia and malaise and urgent referral is needed. This applies especially if there is diplopia or visual loss, because a scan will be required to decide whether surgical intervention is going to be needed to drain an infected sinus.

Lid Tumours

Benign Tumours

Papilloma

Commonly seen on lids near or on margin, may be sessile or pedunculated, sometimes keratinised. It is caused by a virus; easily excised but care must be taken if excision involves the lid margin (Figure 5.12).

Naevus

Flat brown spot on skin, may have hairs, very rarely becomes malignant.

Haemangioma

When seen as red "strawberry mark" at or shortly after birth, may regress completely during first few years of life. Figure 5.13 shows a gross example of the rare cavernous haemangioma, which may be

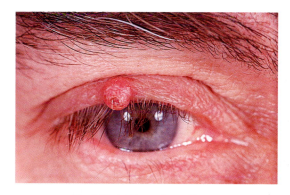

Fig. 5.12.   Lid margin papilloma.

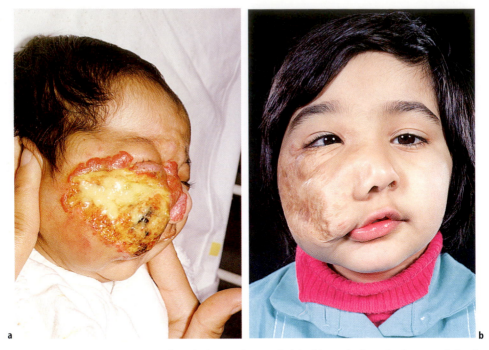

Fig. 5.13. **a** Large disfiguring haemangioma in infancy. **b** The same lesion, which in this case had remained untreated, showing spontaneous regression.

very disfiguring. This also may regress in a remarkable way. "Port wine stain" is the name applied to the capillary haemangioma. This is usually unilateral and when the eyelids are involved there is a risk of association with congenital glaucoma, haemangioma of the choroid and haemangioma of the meninges on the ipselateral side (Sturge–Weber syndrome). Children with port wine stains involving the eyelids need full ophthalmological and neurological examinations.

Dermoid Cyst

Quite commonly seen lump often in or adjacent to eyebrow. Feels cystic and sometimes attached to bone. Present in children as minor cosmetic problem. The cysts are lined by keratinised epithelium and may contain dermal appendages and cholesterol. A scan may be needed before removal since some extend deeply into the skull.

Xanthelasma

Seen as yellowish plaques in skin; usually begin at medial end of lids. Associated rarely with diabetes, hypercholesterolaemia and histiocytosis. Usually no associated systemic disease.

Malignant Tumours

Basal Cell Carcinoma

The most common malignant tumour of the lids, usually on lower lid. Small lump, tends to bleed forming central crust with slightly raised hard

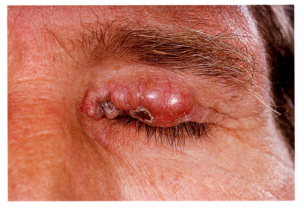

Fig. 5.14. Cystic basal cell carcinoma which has extended to involve most of the upper eyelid.

surround. Tumour is locally invasive only but should be excised to avoid spread into bone. Radiotherapy is effective where local excision is impractical (Figure 5.14).

Squamous Cell Carcinoma

Tends to resemble basal cell carcinoma and biopsy is needed to differentiate. May also be mimicked by a benign self-healing lesion known as keratoacanthoma.

Malignant Melanoma

A raised black pigmented lesion. Highly malignant; rare.

Allergic Disease of the Eyelids

This may present as one of two forms or a mixture of both. The more dramatic is acute allergic blepharitis in which the eyelids swell up rapidly often in response to contact with a plant or eyedrops. The cause must be found and eliminated and treatment with local steroids may be needed. Chronic allergic blepharitis is seen in atopic individuals for example hay fever sufferers or patients with a history of eczema. The diagnosis may require a histological examination of the conjunctival discharge.

Lid Injuries

One of the commonest injuries to the eyelids is due to the presence of a foreign body under the eyelid – a subtarsal foreign body. A small particle of grit lodges near the lower margin of the lid, but to see it the lid must be everted. Every medical student should be familiar with the simple technique of lid eversion. This is performed by gently grasping the lashes of the upper lid between finger and thumb and at the same time placing a glass rod horizontally across the lid. The eyelid is then gently everted by drawing the lid margin upwards and forwards. The manoeuvre is only achieved if the patient is asked to

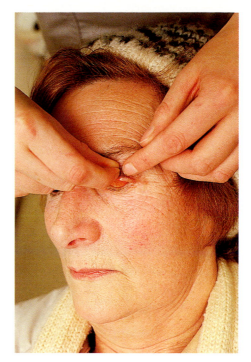

Fig. 5.15.   Everting the upper eyelid.

look down beforehand, and the everted lid is replaced by asking the patient to look upwards. If a small foreign body is seen, it is usually a simple matter to remove it using a cotton-wool bud or even the edge of a clean handkerchief if the former is not available (Figure 5.15).

Cuts on the eyelids may be caused by broken glass or sharp objects such as the ends of screwdrivers. The important thing here is to realise that cuts on the lid margin can leave the patient with a permanently watering eye if not sewn up with proper microscopic control and using very fine sutures. The lids may also be injured by chemical burns or flash burns. Exposure to ultraviolet light, as from a welder's arc or in snow blindness, may cause oedema and erythema of the eyelids. This may appear after an hour or two but resolves spontaneously after about two days.

Common Diseases of the Conjunctiva and Cornea

Subconjunctival Haemorrhage

This is common and tends to occur spontaneously or sometimes after straining, especially vomiting. It may also occur in acute haemorrhagic conjunctivitis due to certain viruses and occasionally bacterial conjunctivitis. The eye becomes suddenly red and although the patient may experience a slight pricking, the condition is usually first noticed in the mirror or by a friend. The haemorrhage gradually absorbs in about 14 days and investigations usually fail to reveal any underlying cause. Very rarely, it is necessary to cauterise the site of bleeding if the haemorrhage is repeated so often that it becomes a nuisance to the patient (Figure 6.1).

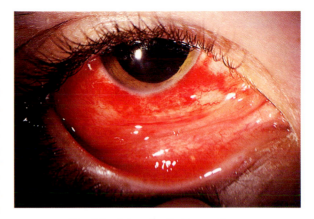

Fig. 6.1. Subconjunctival haemorrhage.

Conjunctivitis

Inflammation of the conjunctiva is extremely common in the general population and the general practitioner is often expected to find out the cause and treat this condition. If we consider that the conjunctiva is a mucous membrane, which is exposed during the waking hours to wind and weather more or less continuously, year in year out, then it is not surprising that this membrane is rather susceptible to inflammation. Furthermore, the conjunctiva can be compared with the lining of a joint, the eye being considered as an unusual type of ball-and-socket joint. The analogy takes on more meaning when the relation between conjunctivitis and some joint disease is seen.

There are a large number of different specific causes of conjunctivitis. Some of these are interesting but rare and it is important that the student obtains an idea of the relative importance and frequency of the different aetiological factors. For this reason, in this chapter a more or less categorical list is given of the different causes. In the chapter on the red eye (Chapter 7) you will find a plan of approach to the red eye which deals with the important and more common causes of conjunctivitis seen in day-to-day practice.

Although the conjunctiva is continuously exposed to infection, it has special protection from the tears, which contain immunoglobulins and lysozyme. The tears also help to wash away debris and foreign bodies and this protective action can explain the self-limiting nature of most types of conjunctivitis.

Symptoms

In all types of conjunctivitis the eye becomes red and feels irritable and gritty as if there were a foreign body under the lid. There is usually some discharge and if marked this may make the eyelids

41

stick together in the mornings. Itchiness may also be present, especially in cases of allergic conjunctivitis. The discharge around the eyelids tends to make vision only intermittently blurred (if at all) and the patient may volunteer that blinking clears the sight.

Signs

Visual acuity is usually normal in conjunctivitis. The conjunctiva appears hyperaemic and there may be evidence of purulent discharge on the lid margins causing matting together of the eyelashes. The redness of the conjunctiva extends to the conjunctival fornices and is usually less marked at the limbus. When a rim of dilated vessels is seen around the cornea, the examiner must suspect a more serious inflammatory reaction within the eye. Apart from being red to a greater or lesser degree, the eyes also tend to water, but a dry eye may lead one to suspect conjunctivitis due to inadequate tear secretion. Drooping of one or both upper lids is a feature of some types of viral conjunctivitis and this may be accompanied by enlargement of the preauricular lymph nodes. Ophthalmologists should train themselves to feel for the preauricular node as a routine part of the examination of such a case. Closer inspection of the conjunctiva may reveal numerous small papillae giving the surface a velvety look, or the papillae may be quite large. Giant papillae under the upper lids are a feature of spring catarrh, a form of allergic conjunctivitis. Close inspection of the conjunctiva may also reveal follicles or lymphoid hyperplasia. Being deep to the epithelium, they are small, pale, raised nodules and are commonly seen in viral conjunctivitis. Follicles under the upper lids are especially characteristic of trachoma.

Microscopy

The examination of a severe case of conjunctivitis of unknown cause is not complete until conjunctival scrapings have been taken. A drop of local anaesthetic is placed in the conjunctival sac and the surface of the conjunctiva at the site of maximal inflammation gently scraped with the blade of a sharp knife or a Kimura spatula. The material obtained is placed on a slide and stained with Gram's stain and Giemsa stain. The infecting organism may thus be revealed or the cell type in the exudate may indicate the underlying cause.

Conjunctival Culture

In most cases of conjunctivitis it may be good medical practice to take a culture from the conjunctival sac and the eyelid margin, but such a measure may not always be possible if a microbiological service is not near to hand. The cultures may be taken with sterile cotton-tipped applicators and sent to the laboratory, in an appropriate medium, as soon as possible.

Causes

- Bacterial.
- Chlamydia.
- Viral.
- Other infective agents.
- Allergic.
- Secondary to lacrimal obstruction corneal disease lid deformities, degenerations, systemic disease.
- Unknown cause.

Bacterial Conjunctivitis

In the UK the commonest organisms to cause conjunctivitis are the pneumococcus, haemophilus and *Staphylococcus aureus*. The last mentioned is normally associated with chronic lid infections, and the acute purulent conjunctivitis, known more familiarly as "pink eye", is usually caused by the pneumococcus. Chronic conjunctivitis may also be caused by *Moraxella lacunata* but this organism is rarely isolated from cases nowadays. An important but rare form of purulent conjunctivitis is that due to *Neisseria gonorrhoeae*; this is still an occasional cause of a severe type of conjunctivitis seen in the new-born babies of infected mothers. Untreated, the cornea also becomes infected, leading to perforation of the globe and permanent loss of vision. Purulent discharge, redness and severe oedema of the eyelids are features of the condition, which is generally known as ophthalmia neonatorum (Figure 6.2). Ophthalmia neonatorum may also be caused by staphylococci and the chlamydia (see inclusion conjunctivitis of the new-born). The disease is notifiable and any infant with purulent discharge from the eyes, particularly between the second and twelfth day *post-partum*, should be suspect. At one time, special blind schools were filled with children who had suffered ophthalmia neonatorum. An active

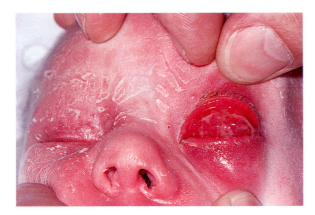

Fig. 6.2. Ophthalmia neonatorium.

campaign against this cause of blindness began at the end of the last century when Carl Crede introduced the principle of careful cleansing of the infant's eyes and the instillation of silver nitrate drops. Blindness from this cause has now disappeared in the UK but there is still a low incidence of ophthalmia neonatorum.

Pink eye is the name given to the type of acute purulent conjunctivitis, which tends to spread rapidly through families or around schools. The eyes begin to itch and within an hour or two produce a sticky discharge, which causes the eyelids to stick together in the mornings. If the disease is mild, it can be treated by cleaning away the discharge with cotton-wool, and it does not usually last longer than three to five days. More severe cases may warrant the prescription of antibiotic drops instilled hourly during the day for three days followed by four times daily for five days. A conjunctival culture should be taken prior to starting treatment. Common-sense precautions against spread of the infection should also be advised, although they are not always successful.

Attempts to culture bacteria from the conjunctival sac of cases of chronic conjunctivitis do not yield much more than commensal organisms.

One particular kind of chronic conjunctivitis in which the inflammation is sited mainly near to the inner and outer canthi is known as angular conjunctivitis with follicles on the superior tarsal conjunctiva. Another feature of this is the excoriation of the skin at the outer canthi from the overflow of infected tears. The clinical picture has been recognised in association with infection by the bacillus *Moraxella lacunata*. Often zinc sulphate drops and the application of zinc cream to the skin at the outer

canthus are sufficient treatment in such cases. Tetracycline ointment may be more effective.

Chlamydia Conjunctivitis

The chlamydia comprise a group of "large viruses" which are sensitive to tetracycline and erythomycin and which cause relatively minor disability to the eyes in northern Europe and the United States when compared to the severe and widespread eye infection seen especially in Africa and the Middle East. Inclusion conjunctivitis ("inclusion blenorrhoea") is the milder form of chlamydial infection and is caused by serotypes D to K of *Chlamydia trachomatis*. The condition tends to be transmitted venereally. The conjunctivitis usually occurs one week after sexual exposure. It may cause a more severe type of conjunctivitis in the new-born child, which can also involve the cornea. The infection is usually self-limiting but has a prolonged course, lasting several months. It responds to treatment with tetracycline. In children and adults tetracycline ointment should be used at least four times daily. In adults the treatment can be supplemented with systemic tetracycline, but the drug should not be used systemically in pregnant mothers or children under seven years of age. The diagnosis depends on the results of conjunctival culture and examination of scrapings and the association of a follicular conjunctivitis with cervicitis or urethritis.

Trachoma

Although a doctor practising in the UK may rarely see a case of trachoma, and even then only in immigrants, it is the commonest cause of blindness in the world and, furthermore, the disease affects about 15% of the world's population. It is spread by direct contact and perpetuated by poverty and unhygienic conditions. Trachoma is caused by *C. trachomatis* serotypes A, B and C and affects underprivileged populations living in conditions of poor hygiene. The disease begins with conjunctivitis, which, instead of resolving, becomes persistent, especially under the upper lid where scarring and distortion of the lid may result. The inflammatory reaction spreads to infiltrate the cornea from above and ultimately the cornea itself may become scarred and opaque (Figure 6.3). At one time trachoma was common in the UK, especially after the Napoleonic wars at the end of the eighteenth century. It had been eliminated by improved hygienic conditions long before the introduction of antibiotics.

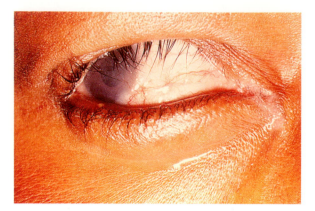

Fig. 6.3. Trachoma trichiasis of upper lid and corneal vascularisation (with acknowledgement to Professor D. Archer).

Adenoviral Conjunctivitis

Acute viral conjunctivitis is common. Several of the adenoviruses may cause it. Usually the eye symptoms follow an upper respiratory tract infection and, although nearly always bilateral, one eye may be infected before the other. The affected eye becomes red and discharges; characteristically the eyelids become thickened and the upper lid may droop. The ophthalmologist's finger should feel for the tell-tale tender enlarged preauricular lymph node. In some cases the cornea becomes involved and subepithelial corneal opacities may appear and persist for several months. If such opacities are situated in the line of sight, the vision may be impaired. There is no known effective treatment but it is usual to treat with an antibiotic drop to prevent secondary infection.

From time to time, epidemics of viral conjunctivitis occur and it is well recognised that spread may result from the use of improperly sterilised ophthalmic instruments or even contaminated solutions of eyedrops, and poor hand-washing techniques.

Herpes Simplex Conjunctivitis

This is usually a unilateral follicular conjunctivitis with preauricular lymph node enlargement. In children it may be the only evidence of primary herpes simplex infection.

Acute Haemorrhagic Conjunctivitis

Acute haemorrhagic conjunctivitis is caused by enterovirus 70 (picornavirus) and usually occurs in epidemics. The disease is hugely contagious but self-limiting.

Other Infective Agents

The conjunctiva may be affected by a wide variety of organisms, some of which are too rare to be considered here, and sometimes the infected conjunctiva is of secondary importance to more severe disease elsewhere in the rest of the body. Molluscum contagiosum is a virus infection, which causes small umbilicated nodules to appear on the skin of the lids and elsewhere on the body, especially the hands. It may be accompanied by conjunctivitis when there are lesions on the lid margin. The infection is usually easily eliminated by curetting each of the lesions. Infection from *Phthirus pubis* (the pubic louse) involving the lashes and lid margins may initially present as conjunctivitis but observation of nits on the lashes should give away the diagnosis.

Allergic Conjunctivitis

Several types of allergic reaction are seen on the conjunctiva and some of these also involve the cornea. They may be listed as follows.

Hay Fever Conjunctivitis

This is simply the commonly experienced red and watering eye that accompanies the sneezing bouts of the hay fever sufferer. The eyes are itchy and mildly infected and there may be conjunctival oedema. If treatment is needed, vasoconstrictors such as, for example, dilute adrenaline or naphazoline drops may be helpful; sodium cromoglycate eyedrops may be used on a more long-term basis. Systemic antihistamines are of limited benefit in controlling the eye changes.

Atopic Conjunctivitis

Unfortunately patients with asthma and eczema may experience recurrent itching and irritation of the conjunctiva. Although atopic conjunctivitis tends to improve over a period of many years, it may result in repeated discomfort and anxiety for the patient, especially as the cornea may become involved, showing a superficial punctate keratitis or, in the worst cases, ulcer formation and scarring.

The diagnosis is usually evident from the history, but conjunctival scrapings show the presence of eosinophils. Patients with atopic keratoconjunctivitis have a higher risk than normal for the development of herpes simplex keratitis; the condition is also associated with the corneal dystrophy known as keratoconus or conical cornea. They are likely to develop skin infections and chronic eyelid infection by staphylococcus. The recurrent itch and irritation (in the absence of infection) is relieved by applying local steroid drops, but in view of the long-term nature of the condition, these should be avoided if possible because of their side-effects. (Local steroids can cause glaucoma in predisposed individuals and aggravate herpes simplex keratitis.)

Vernal Conjunctivitis (Spring Catarrh)

Some children with an atopic history may develop a specific type of conjunctivitis characterised by the presence of giant papillae under the upper lid. The child tends to develop severely watering and itchy eyes in the early spring, which may interfere with schooling. Eversion of the upper lid reveals the raised papillae, which have been likened to cobblestones. In severe cases the cobblestones may coalesce to give rise to giant papillae (Figure 6.4). Occasionally the cornea is also involved initially by punctate keratitis but sometimes it may become vascularised. It is often necessary to treat these cases with local steroids, for example prednisolone drops applied if needed every 2 h for a few days thus enabling the child to return to school. The dose can then be reduced as much as possible down to a maintenance dose over the worst part of the season. Less severe cases may respond well to sodium cromoglycate drops and these may be useful as a long-term measure; it is useful in preventing but not in controlling acute exacerbations.

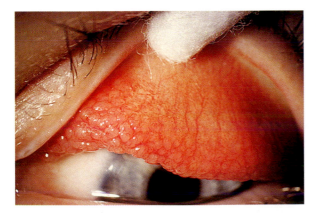

Fig. 6.4. Vernal conjunctivitis (spring catarrh) papillary reaction.

Secondary Conjunctivitis

Inflammation of the conjunctiva may often be secondary to other more important primary pathology. The following are some of the possible underlying causes of this type of conjunctivitis:

- Lacrimal obstruction
- corneal disease
- lid deformities
- degenerations
- systemic disease.

Lacrimal obstruction may cause recurrent unilateral purulent conjunctivitis and it is important to consider this possibility in recalcitrant cases because early resolution may be achieved simply by syringing the tear ducts. Corneal ulceration from a variety of causes is often associated with conjunctivitis and here the treatment is aimed primarily at the cornea. Occasionally the presence of one of the two common acquired lid deformities, entropion and ectropion, may be the underlying cause. Sometimes the diagnosis may be missed, especially in the case of entropion when the deformity is not present all the time. Other lid deformities may also have the same effect. A special type of degenerative change is seen in the conjunctiva, which is more marked in hot, dry, dusty climates. It appears that the combination of lid movement in blinking, dryness and dustiness of the atmosphere and perhaps some abnormal factor in the patient's tears or tear production may lead to the heaping up of subconjunctival yellow elastic tissue which is often infiltrated with lymphocytes. The lesion is seen as a yellow plaque on the conjunctiva in the exposed area of the bulbar conjunctiva and usually on the nasal side. Such early degenerative changes are extremely common in all climates as a natural ageing phenomenon, but under suitable conditions the heaped-up tissue spreads into the cornea, drawing a triangular band of conjunctiva with it. The eye becomes irritable due to associated conjunctivitis and in worst cases the degenerative plaque extends across the cornea and affects the vision. The early stage of the condition, which is common and limited to a small area of the conjunctiva, is termed a pingueculum and the more advanced lesion spreading onto the cornea is known as a pterygium (Figure 6.5). Pterygium is more common in Africa, India, Australia, China and the Middle East than in Europe. It is rarely seen in white races living in temperate climates. Treatment is by surgical excision if the cornea is significantly affected with progression towards the visual axis; antibiotic

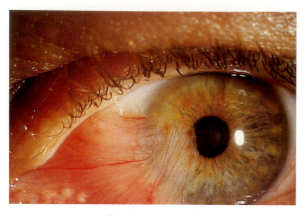

Fig. 6.5.   Pterygium.

drops may be required if the conjunctiva is infected. Non-infective inflammation of pterygium is treated with topical steroids.

Finally, when considering secondary causes of conjunctivitis one must be aware that redness and congestion of the conjunctiva with secondary infection may be an indicator of systemic disease. Examples of this are the red eye of renal failure and gout and also polycythaemia rubra. The association

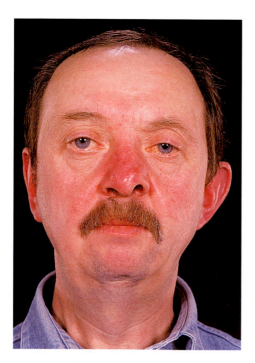

Fig. 6.6.   Acne rosacea.

of conjunctivitis, arthritis and non-specific urethritis makes up the triad of Reiter's syndrome. Some diseases cause abnormality of the tears and these have already been discussed with dry eye syndromes, the most common being rheumatoid arthritis. However there are other rarer diseases which upset the quality or production of tears such as sarcoidosis, pemphigus and Stevens–Johnson syndrome. Thyrotoxicosis is a more common systemic disease which is associated with conjunctivitis, but the other eye signs such as lid retraction, conjunctival oedema and proptosis are usually more evident. A rather persistent type of conjunctivitis is seen in patients with acne rosacea. Here, the diagnosis is usually, but not always, made evident by the appearance of the skin of the nose, cheeks and forehead, but the corneal lesions of rosacea are also quite characteristic (Figure 6.6). The cornea becomes invaded from the periphery by wedge-shaped tongues of blood vessels associated with recurrent corneal ulceration. Rosacea keratoconjunctivitis is seen less commonly now, perhaps because it responds well to treatment with local and systemic tetracycline, a treatment that has now largely replaced the use of local steroids.

Corneal Foreign Body

Small particles of grit or dust very commonly become embedded in the cornea and every casualty officer is aware of the increasing incidence of this occurrence on windy, dry days. Small foreign bodies also become embedded as the result of using high-speed grinding tools without adequate eye protection. The dentist's drill may also be a source of foreign bodies, but the most troublesome are those particles that have been heated by grinding or chiselling. It is important to have some understanding of the anatomy of the cornea if one is attempting to remove a corneal foreign body. One must realise, for example, that the surface epithelium can be stripped off from the underlying layer and can regrow and fill raw areas with extreme rapidity. Under suitable conditions the whole surface epithelium can reform in about 48 h. The layer underlying or posterior to the surface epithelium is known as Bowman's membrane and if this layer is damaged by the injury or cut into unnecessarily by over-zealous use of surgical instruments, then a permanent scar may be left in the cornea. When the epithelium alone is involved there is usually no scar, and healing results in perfect restoration of the optical properties of the surface.

The stroma of the cornea is surprisingly tough, permitting some degree of boldness when removing deeply embedded foreign bodies. It should be remembered that if the cornea has been perforated, then the risk of intraocular infection or loss of aqueous dictates that the wound should be repaired under full sterile conditions in the operating theatre.

Signs and Symptoms

Patients usually know when a foreign body has gone into their eye and the history is clear cut – but not always. Occasionally the complaint is simply a red sore eye, which may have been present for some time. Spotting these corneal foreign bodies is really lesson number one in ocular examination. It involves employing the important basic principles of examining the anterior segment of the eye. Most foreign bodies can be seen without the use of the slit-lamp microscope if the eye is examined carefully and with a focused beam of light. Figure 6.7 demonstrates the great advantage of the focused beam, and in fact this very principle is used in slit-lamp microscopy. If the foreign body has been present for any length of time, there will be a ring of ciliary injection around the cornea due to the dilatation of the deeper episcleral capillaries, which lie near the corneal margin. Ciliary injection is a sure warning sign of corneal or intraocular pathology.

Treatment

The aim of treatment is, of course, to remove the foreign body completely. Sometimes this is not as easy as it may seem, especially when a hot metal particle lies embedded in a "rust ring". In instances when it is clear that much digging is going to be needed, it may be prudent to leave the rust ring for 24 h, after which it becomes easier to remove. The procedure for removing a foreign body should be as follows: the patient lies down on a couch or dental chair and one or two drops of proparacaine hydrochloride 0.5% (Ophthaine) or a similar local anaesthetic are instilled on the affected eye. A good light on a stand is needed, preferably one with a focused beam and the eyelids are held open with a speculum (Figure 6.8). The doctor will also usually require some optical aid in the form of special magnifying spectacles, for example "Bishop Harman's glasses" or the slit-lamp. Many foreign bodies can be easily removed with a cotton-wool bud and his should always be tried first. If this fails, a blunt spud may succeed. When the foreign body is more deeply

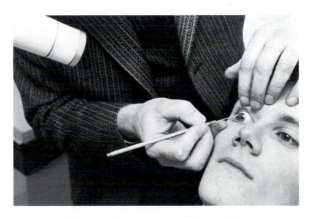

Fig. 6.8. Removing corneal foreign body.

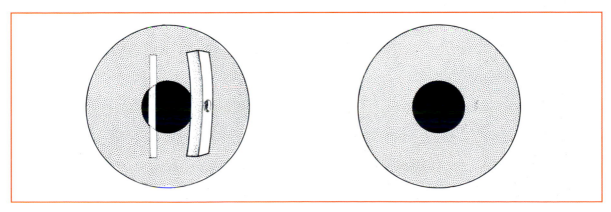

Fig. 6.7. Focal illumination of corneal foreign body.

embedded, it will be necessary to pick it off with a sharp pointed instrument such as a scalpel blade or a hypodermic needle. There are a variety of instruments specially designed for this purpose. Once the foreign body has been removed, an antibiotic drop is placed in the eye and the speculum is withdrawn. The lids are then splinted together by means of a firm pad. There is no doubt that the corneal epithelium heals more quickly if the eyelids are splinted in this way. It is usually advisable to see the patient the following day if possible to make sure that all is well, and if the damaged spot on the cornea is no longer staining with fluorescein, the pad can be left off. Antibiotic drops should be continued at least three times daily for a few days after the cornea has healed. The visual acuity of the patient should always be checked before final discharge.

There are one or two factors that should always be borne in mind when treating patients with corneal foreign bodies: in most instances healing takes place without any problem but, very rarely, the vision may be permanently impaired by scarring. Also on very rare occasions, the site of corneal damage becomes infected and if neglected the infection may enter the eye and cause endophthalmitis with total blindness of the affected eye. This is a well-recognised tragedy, which should never happen in an age of antibiotics. Of course, if the eye has been perforated, endophthalmitis is a more or less inevitable sequel in the absence of antibiotic treatment. One only has to examine old hospital case notes from the pre-antibiotic era to obtain proof of this.

Let us remember that a perforating injury of the eye is a surgical emergency. Any doubt about the possibility of a perforating injury of the cornea can usually be resolved by examining it carefully with the slit-lamp microscope. One other factor to bear in mind is the possibility of a retained intraocular foreign body. Sometimes the patient may be quite unaware of such an injury and this may mislead the doctor into underestimating the serious nature of the problem. The answer for the doctor is "when in doubt, X-ray", especially when a hammer and chisel or high-speed drill have been used. A retained intraocular foreign body may not set up an inflammatory reaction or irreversible degenerative changes until several weeks or even months have elapsed (Figure 6.9).

Corneal Ulceration

Corneal ulcers may arise spontaneously (primary) or they may result from some defect in the normal protective mechanism or sometimes they are part of a more generalised susceptibility to infection (secondary). The nerve endings in the cornea are pain-sensitive endings and a light touch is felt as a sharp pain. Furthermore, stimulation of these nerves causes a vigorous blink reflex and the eye begins to water excessively. A very effective protective mechanism is therefore brought into action, which tends to clear away infection or foreign bodies and warns the patient of trouble. In most instances of corneal ulceration the eye is painful, photophobic and waters. The conjunctiva is usually injected and there may be ciliary injection.

Types of Corneal Ulcer

Due to Direct Trauma

The corneal epithelium becomes disrupted and abraded by certain characteristic injuries. It is surprising how the same old story keeps repeating itself: the mother caught in the eye by the child's fingernail, the edge of a newspaper, the backlash from the branch of a tree. The injury is excruciatingly painful and the symptoms are often made much worse by the rapid eye movements of an anxious patient and sometimes by vigorous rubbing

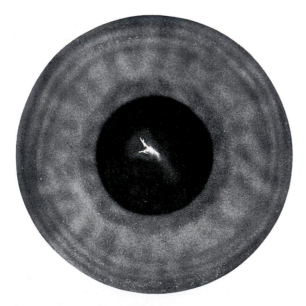

Fig. 6.9. Beware of the full thickeness corneal scar, when in doubt do an X-ray.

of the eye. The patient complains that there is something in the eye and once the diagnosis has been made it may be difficult to persuade the patient that there is no foreign body. A denuded area of cornea is seen which stains with fluorescein. It may not be possible to examine the patient until a drop of local anaesthetic has been instilled into the eye, but, as a general rule, local anaesthetic drops should not be used to treat "sore eye". This is because healing is impaired and serious damage to the eye may result. Anaesthetic drops should only be used as a single-dose diagnostic measure in such cases. Treatment involves the instillation of a mydriatic such as homatropine 1% and an antibiotic ointment such as chloramphenicol 0.5% after which special care is needed to fix the eyelids. This is probably best achieved by directly sticking the eyelids together with two vertically placed short strips of micropore surgical tape. A pad is then placed over the closed eyelids. The patient is then given some analgesic tablets to take home and is advised to rest quietly until the eye is inspected the following day. The pad can be left off once the epithelium has healed over, but even then the patient should continue to instil an antibiotic ointment in the eye at night for several weeks. The reason for taking a little trouble over the management of a patient with a corneal abrasion is the recurrent nature of the condition. All too often after some months or even a few years, the patient begins to experience a sharp pain in the injured eye on waking in the morning. It is as if the cornea, or the weak part of the cornea, becomes stuck to the posterior surface of the upper lid during the night. The pain wears off after an hour or two and when the patient presents to the doctor there may be no obvious cause for the symptoms. In actual fact careful examination with the slit-lamp reveals very minute cysts or white specks at the site of the original abrasion, indicating a weak area of attachment of the corneal epithelium. Severe recurrent corneal abrasion is best dealt with in an eye department where slit-lamp control is available.

Due to Bacteria

The commonest ulcer of this type is known as a "marginal ulcer". The patient complains of a persistently red eye, which is moderately sore. Examination reveals conjunctival congestion, which is often mainly localised to an area adjacent to the corneal ulcer. The ulcer is seen as a white spot near the corneal margin but there is usually a small gap of clear cornea between it and the limbus (the cor-

neoscleral junction). Such marginal ulcers are thought to be due to exotoxins from *Staphylococcus aureus*, mainly because they are often associated with *S. aureus blepharitis*. On the other hand, it is not possible to grow the organism from the corneal lesion, and for this reason it is said that the infiltrated area is some form of allergic response to the infecting organism. Furthermore, these marginal ulcers respond very rapidly to treatment with a steroid–antibiotic mixture. It is essential that the usual precautions before applying local steroids to the eye are taken, that is to say, the possibility of herpes simplex infection should be excluded and the intraocular pressure should be monitored if the treatment is to continue on a more long-term basis.

A wide range of other bacteria are known to cause corneal ulceration, but, by and large, infections only occur as a secondary problem when the defences of the cornea are impaired, for example, underlying corneal disease (trauma bullous keratopathy), dry eyes or contact lens wear.

There are three bacteria, which can produce corneal infection despite healthy epithelium: *Neisseria gonorrhoea*, meningitis and diphtheria. Pathogens most often associated with corneal infections, however, are *Staphylococcus aureus*, *S. pneumoniae*, *Pseudomonas aeruginosa* and the enterobacteria (*Escherichia coli*, *Proteus* sp., and *Klebsiella* sp.). Pseudomonas is an especially virulent bacterium as it can cause rapid corneal perforation if inadequately treated.

Usually there is pain, photophobia, watering and discharge in addition to redness. Examination reveals ciliary injection and a corneal defect, which may have a greyish base (infiltration). There is most often an associated (secondary) iritis, which may be severe giving rise to a hypopyon (layer of pus in the anterior chamber).

Bacterial corneal ulcers are sight threatening and require urgent treatment. The causative organism needs to be identified by corneal scrapes. Appropriate antibiotics usually a combination of gentamicin and cefuroxime applied frequently in hospital provides a broad spectrum until the organisms are identified.

Due to Acanthamoeba

Acanthamoeba are a free-living genus of amoeba that has been increasingly associated with keratitis. The keratitis is usually chronic and may follow minor trauma. Contact lens wearers are particularly at risk of this infection.

Due to Viruses

Apart from other rare types of virus infection, there is one outstanding example of this – herpes simplex keratitis. The condition seems to be more common than it used to be, perhaps because the incidence of other types of corneal ulcer has become less with the more liberal use of local antibiotics on the eye. Every eye casualty department has a few patients with this debilitating condition, which may put a patient off work for many months. Fortunately it is only a few cases that cause such a problem, and most instances of this common condition give rise to a week or 10 days of incapacity. Herpes simplex is thought to produce a primary infection in infants and younger children, which is transferred from the lips of the mother and may be subclinical. Sometimes a vesicular rash develops around the eyelids accompanied by fever and enlargement of the preauricular lymph nodes. Whatever the initial

manifestation of primary infection, it is thought that many members of the population harbour the virus in a latent form so that overt infection in an adult tends to appear in association with other illnesses. Most people are familiar with the cold sores that appear on the lips due to herpes simplex. Sometimes, after a cold, one eye becomes sore and irritable and inspection of the cornea shows the very characteristic corneal changes of herpes simplex infection. A slightly raised granular, star-shaped or dendriform lesion is seen which takes up fluorescein (Figure 6.10a). The virus can be cultivated from this lesion and the size of the dendriform figure is some guide to prognosis. A large lesion extending across the cornea, especially across the optical axis (i.e. the centre of the cornea), is likely to be the one which is going to give trouble and it is better that the patient should be warned about it at this stage. After a few days, or sometimes weeks, the epithelial lesion heals

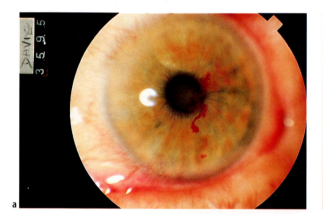

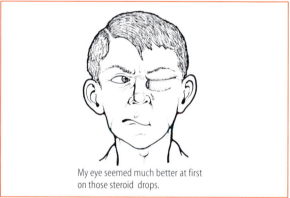

My eye seemed much better at first on those steroid drops.

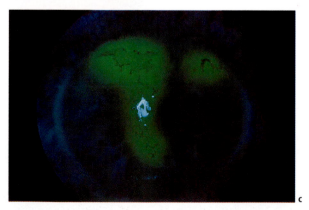

Fig. 6.10.   **a** Dendritic ulcer of cornea. **b** Use of steroid drops in herpes simplex keratitis. **c** Progression of herpes simplex keratitis following use of steroid eye drops (with acknowledgement to Professor H. Dua).

and at this point complete resolution may occur or an inflammatory reaction may appear in the stroma deep to the infected epithelium. The eye remains red and irritable to an incapacitating degree and further dendritic ulcers may subsequently appear. In worse cases the cornea may become anaesthetic so that although the eye may be more comfortable, the problems of a numb cornea are added to the original condition. Healing tends to occur with a vascular scar.

Treatment of Herpes Simplex Keratitis

Antiviral agents are usually the first line of treatment. Examples of currently used antiviral agents are idoxuridine, trifluorothymidine, cytarabine and acyclovir. The most effective is acyclovir. Unfortunately none of these agents is curative, but they are thought to have some effect on acute rather than chronic cases. Early diagnosis and treatment seem to give the best chance of avoiding recurrences. The removal of virus-containing epithelial cells (debridement) is now indicated only in cases that are resistant to antiviral agents, where there is toxicity to the drugs, or there is difficulty in acquiring or applying the antiviral agents. An antibiotic drop and cycloplegic are instilled and a firm pad and bandage applied. Touching the debrided area with iodine is now obsolete. Following this procedure the eye may become very sore and the patient is given an analgesic. Often the corneal epithelium will heal after 48 h and the condition will be cured. Larger ulcers may not respond very satisfactorily to this treatment. Steroids should not be used in the treatment of dendritic ulcers of the cornea (Figure 6.10b). It is well recognised that steroid drops enhance the replication of the herpes simplex virus (Figure 6.10c). They reduce the local inflammatory reaction and may give the false impression that the eye is improving. However, persistent use of local steroids in such cases may result in corneal thinning and even corneal perforation. Once the dendritic ulcer has healed, residual stromal infiltration is then sometimes treated by carefully gauged doses of steroids, but this should be under strict ophthalmological supervision. In more severe cases, secondary iritis or secondary glaucoma may complicate the picture and require special treatment. The decision whether or not to apply a pad to the eye depends on the state of the corneal epithelium and also on the patient's response. In the worst cases it may be advisable to perform a tarsorrhaphy, that is to say, the lids are stitched together in such a way that they remain closed when the stitches are removed. An alternative is to induce drooping of the eyelid by an injection of botulinum toxin into the levator muscle. Surprisingly, the keratitis seems to heal usually in one to two weeks when this is done and the patient may be able to return to work providing the work does not require the use of both eyes. When herpetic keratitis has taken its toll leaving a scarred cornea, the sight may eventually be restored again by a corneal graft. Unfortunately, recurrences still often occur and dendritic ulcers may appear on the graft.

Due to Damage to the Corneal Nerve Supply

When the ophthalmic division of the trigeminal nerve is damaged by disease or injury, the cornea may become numb and there is a high risk of corneal ulceration. Such neurotrophic ulcers are characteristically painless and easily become infected, with possible disastrous results. A tarsorrhaphy may be needed to save the eye but sometimes a soft contact lens may suffice provided the ulcer is not infected at the time. Before embarking on the treatment of an anaesthetic cornea, the cause should be established and this may involve a full neurological investigation.

Due to Exposure

When the normal "windscreen wiper" mechanism of the lids is faulty, as, for example when the eyelids have been injured or in a case of facial palsy, then the surface of the cornea may dry and become ulcerated. The same problem occurs in the unconscious patient unless great care is taken to keep the eyelids closed. Most cases of Bell's palsy recover sufficiently quickly to prevent exposure keratitis, but when severe and when recovery is poor, a tarsorrhaphy, or at least treatment with an eyepad and local antibiotic ointment at night, may be needed. It is important to bear in mind that the same risk is evident in patients with severe thyrotoxic exophthalmos.

Corneal Dystrophies

There are a number of specific corneal dystrophies, most of which are inherited and most of which cannot be diagnosed without the aid of the slit-lamp microscope. For this reason they will not be dealt with in any detail here. A list for reference is given in Table 6.1.

Table 6.1.   Corneal dystrophies

Anterior dystrophies (corneal epithelium and Bowman's membrane):
 Microcystic
 Reis Buckler's

Stromal dystrophies:
 lattice
 macular
 granular

Posterior dystrophies (corneal endothelium and Descemet's membrane):
 Fuch's
 posterior polymorphous

Ectatic dystrophies:
 keratoconus
 keratoglobus

Keratoconus (or conical cornea) is perhaps the commonest. It is still rare in the general population but is familiar to general practitioners looking after student populations because it tends to appear in this age group. The condition is bilateral and may be inherited as an autosomal recessive trait, although most patients do not have a positive family history. It should be suspected in patients who show a rapid change of refractive error, particularly if a large amount of myopic astigmatism suddenly appears. Often, but not always, there is an associated history of asthma and hay fever. The cornea shows central thinning and protrudes anteriorly. This may be observed with the naked eye by asking the patient to sit down and then standing behind him so that one can look down on his downturned eye. By holding up the upper lids one can make an estimate of the abnormal shape of the cornea by noting how the cornea shapes the lower lid. Alternatively, the patient's cornea can be observed using Placido's disc. This ingenious instrument is simply a disc with a hole in the centre of it through which one observes the patient's cornea. On the patient's side of the disc is a series of concentric circles which can be seen by the observer reflected on the patient's cornea (Figure 6.11). Distortion of these circles indicates the abnormal shape of the cornea. Of course, more accurate assessment of the cornea can be made by observing it with the slit-lamp microscope and still more information can be obtained by keratometry or corneal topography, that is, using an instrument to measure the curvature of the cornea in different meridians. Keratoconus tends to progress slowly and contact lenses may be very helpful. Sometimes a corneal graft is required. Less common corneal dystrophies include Fuch's endothelial, stromal and anterior dystrophies.

Corneal Degenerations

Apart from the inherited corneal dystrophies, certain changes are often seen in the cornea with ageing such as arcus senilis and endothelial pigmentation. Band degeneration refers to a deposition of calcium salts in the anterior layers of the cornea. The calcification is first seen at the margin of the cornea in the nine o'clock and three o'clock area, but it may gradually extend across the normally exposed part of the cornea. It is seen in cases of chronic

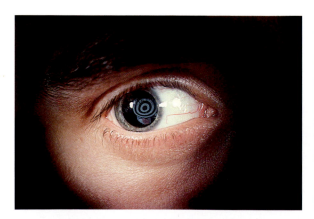

Fig. 6.11.   Keratoconus; placido disc image.

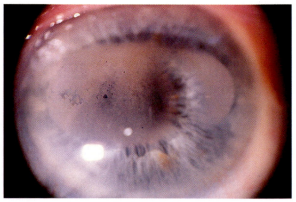

Fig. 6.12.   Band keratopathy.

iridocyclitis, in particular in patients with juvenile rheumatoid arthritis and also in those with sarcoidosis. In fact, band degeneration is seen in any eye, which has become degenerate or in cases of long-standing corneal disease (Figure 6.12). Although band degeneration can, if sufficiently advanced, be diagnosed quite easily with the naked eye, most degenerative conditions of the cornea can only be diagnosed and classified under the microscope. Other corneal degenerations include Salzmann's nodular dystrophy and lipid keratopathies

Corneal Oedema

To the naked eye, corneal oedema may not be very obvious but careful inspection will reveal a lack of lustre when the affected cornea is compared with that on the other side. The normal sparkle of the eye is no longer evident and the iris becomes less well defined. Microscopically a bedewed appearance is seen, minute droplets being evident in the epithelium. When the stroma is also involved this may seem misty and may be also infiltrated with inflammatory cells which are seen as powdery white dots. When the oedema is long-standing the droplets in the epithelium coalesce to produce blisters or bullae.

The more important causes of corneal oedema are as follows.

- acute narrow angle glaucoma
- virus keratitis
- trauma
- contact lenses
- postoperative
- Fuch's endothelial dystrophy.

When the intraocular pressure is suddenly raised from any cause, the cornea becomes oedematous. The normal cornea needs to be relatively dehydrated in order to maintain its transparency, and the necessary level of dehydration seems to depend on active removal of water by the corneal endothelium as well as an adequate oxygen supply from the tears. The mechanism is impaired not only by raising the intraocular pressure, but also by infection or trauma. Senile degenerative changes may also be the sole underlying cause due to failure of the endothelial pumping mechanisms. Contact lenses, if ill fitting and worn for too long a period, may prevent adequate oxygen reaching the cornea, with resulting oedema. The management of corneal oedema depends on the management of the underlying cause. Oedema due to endothelial damage may respond in its early stages to local steroids and sometimes a clear cornea may be maintained by the use of osmotic agents such as hypertonic saline or glycerol. Chronic corneal oedema tends to be painful and often acute episodes of pain occur when bullae rupture leaving exposed corneal nerves. In such cases it may be necessary to consider a tarsorrhaphy, or in some instances a corneal graft may prove beneficial. The pain of corneal oedema is a late symptom and in its early stages oedema simply causes blurring of the vision and the appearance of coloured haloes around light bulbs. This is simply a "bathroom window" effect. Patients with cataracts also see haloes, so that defects in other parts of the optical media of the eye may give a similar effect.

Absent Corneal Sensation

Corneal sensation is supplied by the fifth nerve. About 70 nerve fibres are present in the superficial layers of the cornea and they can often be seen when the cornea is examined with the slit-lamp microscope. They appear as white threads running mainly radially. Asking the patient to gaze straight ahead then lightly touching the cornea with a fine wisp of cotton-wool can assess corneal anaesthesia. Care must be taken not to touch the lid margins when doing this. The blink reflex is then noted and it is also important to ask the patient what has been felt. In the case of elderly people the blink reflex may be reduced, but a slight prick should be evident when the cornea is touched. Attempts to quantify corneal anaesthesia have led to the development of graded strengths of bristle, which can be applied to the cornea instead of cotton-wool.

Corneal anaesthesia may result from a lesion at any point in the Vth cranial nerve from the cornea to the brainstem. In the cornea itself, herpes simplex infection may ultimately result in anaesthesia. Herpes zoster is especially liable to lead to this problem and, because this condition may often be treated at home rather than in the ward, it will be considered in more detail here.

Herpes Zoster Ophthalmicus

This is due to the varicella–zoster virus, the same virus that causes chickenpox. It is thought that the initial infection with the virus occurs with an attack of childhood chickenpox and that the virus remains in the body in a latent form, subsequently to manifest itself as herpes zoster in some individuals. The virus appears to lodge in the Gasserian ganglion. The onset of the condition is heralded by headache and the appearance of one or two vesicles on the forehead. Over the next three or four days the vesicles multiply and appear on the distribution of one or all of the branches of the Vth cranial nerve. The patient may develop a temperature and usually experiences malaise and considerable pain. Sometimes a chickenpox-like rash appears over the rest of the body. The eye itself is most at risk when the upper division of the Vth nerve is involved. There may be vesicles on the lids and conjunctiva and, when the cornea is affected, punctate-staining areas are seen which become minute subepithelial opacities. After four days to a week, the infection reaches its peak; the eyelids on the affected side may be closed by swelling, and oedema of the lids may spread across to the other eye (Figure 6.13). The vesicles become pustular and then form crusts

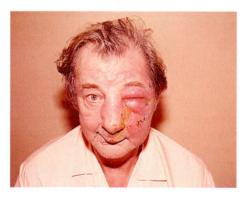

Fig. 6.13.   herpes zoster ophthalmicus.

which are then shed over a period of two or three weeks. In most cases complete resolution occurs with remarkably little scarring of the skin considering the appearance in the acute stage. However, the cornea may be rendered permanently anaesthetic and the affected area of skin produces annoying paraesthesiae, amounting quite often to persistent rather severe neuralgia which may dog the patient for many years. Other complications include extraocular muscle palsies or rarely, encephalitis. Iridocyclitis is fairly common and glaucoma may develop and lead to blindness if untreated. At present there is no known effective treatment other than the use of local steroids and acyclovir for the uveitis, and acetazolamide or topical b-blockers for the glaucoma. Administration of systemic acyclovir early in the disease is thought to reduce the neuralgia. The disease has to run its course and the patient, who is usually elderly, may require much support and advice, especially when post-herpetic neuralgia is severe. It is accepted practice to treat the eye at risk with antibiotic drops and a weak mydriatic. Analgesics are, of course, also usually needed, often on a long-term basis.

Other causes of corneal anaesthesia include surgical division of the Vth cranial nerve for trigeminal neuralgia or any space-occupying lesion along the nerve pathway. The possibility of exposure and drying of the cornea must always be borne in mind in the unconscious or the anaesthetised patient since corneal ulceration and infection will soon result if this is neglected.

Corneal anaesthesia due to nerve damage is nearly always permanent and, if it is complete, it may often be necessary to protect the eye by means of a tarsorrhaphy or botulinum toxin. Lesser degrees of corneal anaesthesia may be treated by instilling an antibiotic ointment at night and, if a more severe punctate keratitis develops, by padding the eye.

The Red Eye 7

Redness of the eye is one of the commonest signs in ophthalmology, being a feature of a wide range of ophthalmological conditions, some of which are severe and sight threatening whereas some are mild and of little consequence. Occasionally the red eye may be the first sign of important systemic disease. It is important that every practising doctor has an understanding of the differential diagnosis of this common sign, and a categorisation of the signs, symptoms and management of the red eye will now be made from the standpoint of the non-specialist general practitioner.

The simplest way of categorising these patients is in terms of their visual acuity. As a general rule, if the sight, as measured on the Snellen test chart, is impaired, then the cause may be more serious. The presence or absence of pain is also of significance but as this depends in part on the pain threshold of the subject, it may be a misleading symptom. Disease of the conjunctiva alone is not usually painful whereas disease of the cornea or iris is generally very painful.

The red eye will therefore be considered under two headings: the red eye, which sees well and is not painful, and the red eye, which does not see well and is acutely painful.

Red Eye Which Is Not Painful and Sees Normally

Subconjunctival Haemorrhage

Careful examination of the eye will easily confirm that its redness is due to blood rather than dilated blood vessels, and the redness may be noticed by someone other than the patient. The condition is common and resolves in about 10–14 days. It is extremely unusual for a blood dyscrasia to present with subconjunctival haemorrhages. Although vomiting or a bleeding tendency may also be rare causes, the normal practice is to reassure the patient rather than embark on extensive investigations, because the majority of cases are due to spontaneous bleeding from a conjunctival capillary. This may be spontaneous and can result from a sudden increase in venous pressure, for example after coughing.

Conjunctivitis

Examination of the eye reveals inflammation, that is, dilatation of the conjunctival capillaries and larger blood vessels, associated with more or less discharge from the eye. The exact site of the inflammation should be noted and it is especially useful to note whether the deeper capillaries around the margin of the cornea are involved. The resulting pink flush encircling the cornea is called "ciliary injection" and is a warning of corneal or intraocular inflammation. For clinical purposes it is useful to divide conjunctivitis into acute and chronic types.

Acute

This is usually infective and due to a bacterium; it is more common in young people. It may spread rapidly through families or schools without serious consequence other than a few days' incapacity. When adults develop acute conjunctivitis it is worth searching for a possible underlying cause, especially a blocked tear duct when the condition is unilateral. Sometimes an ingrowing lash may be the cause or occasionally a free-floating eyelash lodges in the lacrimal punctum. The important symptoms of acute conjunctivitis are redness, irritation and sticking together of the eyelids in the mornings. Management entails finding the cause and using antibiotic drops if the symptoms are severe enough to warrant this. However, it must be remembered that the inadequate and intermittent use of antibiotic eyedrops may simply encourage growth of resistant organisms.

Chronic

This is a very common cause of the red eye and almost a daily problem in non-specialised ophthalmic practice. If we consider that the conjunctiva is a mucous membrane which is daily exposed to the elements, it is perhaps not surprising that after many years it tends to become chronically inflamed and irritable. The frequency and nuisance value of the symptoms are reflected in the large across-the-counter sales of various eyewashes and solutions aimed at relieving "eye strain" or "tired eyes". The symptoms of chronic conjunctivitis are therefore redness and irritation of the eyes with a minimal degree of discharge and sticking of the lids. If there is an allergic background, itching may also be a main feature. The chronically inflamed conjunctiva accumulates minute particles of calcium salts within the mucous glands. These conjunctival concretions are shed from time to time producing a feeling of grittiness. When confronted with such a patient there are a number of key symptoms to be elicited and these can be related to a checklist of causes mentioned below.

Key Symptoms

● Environmental factors, especially eyedrops, make-up or foreign bodies.
● Lids stick in mornings?
● Do the eyes itch?
● Emotional stress or psychiatric illness?

Checklist of Causes

● Eyelids. Deformities such as entropion or ectropion.
● Displaced eyelashes.
● Chronic blepharitis.
● Refractive error. A proportion of patients who have never worn glasses and need them or who are wearing incorrectly prescribed or out-of-date glasses present with the features of chronic con-

junctivitis, the symptoms being relieved by the proper use of spectacles. The cause is not clear but possibly related to rubbing the eyes.
● Dry eye syndrome. The possibility of a defect in the secretion of tears or mucus can only be confirmed by more elaborate tests, but this should be suspected in patients with rheumatoid arthritis or sarcoidosis.
● Foreign body. Contact lenses and mascara particles are the commonest foreign bodies to cause chronic conjunctivitis.
● Stress. Often a period of stress seems to be closely related to the symptoms and perhaps eye rubbing is also the cause in these patients.
● Allergy. It is very unusual to be able to incriminate a specific allergen for chronic conjunctivitis, unlike allergic blepharitis. On the other hand, hay fever and asthma may be the background cause.
● Infection. Chronic conjunctivitis may begin as an acute infection, usually viral and usually following an upper respiratory tract infection.
● Drugs. The long-term use of adrenaline drops may cause dilatation of the conjunctival vessels and irritation in the eye. In 1974 it was shown that the β-blocking drug practolol (since withdrawn from the market) could cause a severe dry eye syndrome in rare instances. Since then there have been several reports of mild reactions to other available β-blockers, although such reactions are difficult to distinguish from chronic conjunctivitis from other causes.
● Systemic causes. Congestive cardiac failure, renal failure, Reiter's disease, polycythaemia, gout, rosacea as well as other causes of orbital venous congestion such as orbital tumours may all cause vascular congestion and irritation of the conjunctiva. Migraine may also be associated with redness of the eye on one side and chronic alcoholism is a cause of bilateral conjunctival congestion.

Episcleritis

Sometimes the eye becomes red due to inflammation of the connective tissue underlying the conjunctiva, that is, the episclera. The condition may be localised or diffuse. There is no discharge and the eye is uncomfortable although not usually painful. The condition responds to sodium salicylate given systemically and to the administration of local steroids or non-steroid anti-inflammatory agents. The underlying cause is often never discovered, although there is a well-recognised link with the col-

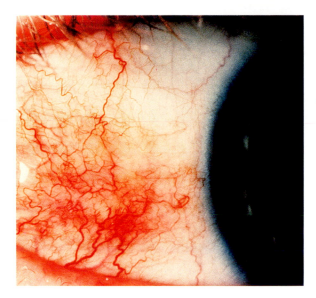

Fig. 7.1. Episcleritis (with acknowledgement to Professor H. Dua).

lagen and dermatological diseases, especially acne rosacea. Episcleritis tends to recur and may persist for several weeks producing a worrying cosmetic blemish in a young person (Figure 7.1).

Red Painful Eye Which May See Normally

Scleritis

Inflammation of the sclera is a less common cause of the red eye. There is no discharge but the eye is painful. Vision is usually normal, unless the inflammation involves the posterior sclera. It is most often seen in association with rheumatoid arthritis and other collagen diseases and sometimes may become severe and progressive to the extent of causing perforation of the globe. For this reason steroids must be administered with extreme care. Treatment normally is with systemically administered non-steroidal anti-inflammatory agents, for example, flurbeprofen (Froben) tablets.

Red Painful Eye Which Cannot See

It is worth emphasising again that the red painful eye with poor vision is likely to be a serious problem, often requiring urgent admission to hospital or at least intensive outpatient treatment as a sight-saving measure. The following are the principal causes.

Acute Glaucoma

The important feature here is that acute glaucoma occurs in long-sighted people and there is usually a previous history of headaches and seeing haloes round lights in the evenings. The raised intraocular pressure damages the iris sphincter and for this reason the pupil is semidilated. Oedema of the cornea causes the eye to lose its lustre and gives the iris a hazy appearance (Figure 7.2). The eye is extremely tender and painful and the patient may be nauseated and vomiting. Immediate admission to hospital is essential where the intraocular pressure is first controlled medically and then bilateral laser iridotomies or surgical peripheral iridectomies performed to relieve pupil block. Mydriatics should not be given to patients with suspected narrow angle glaucoma, without consultation with an ophthalmologist

Acute Iritis

The eye is painful, especially when attempting to view near objects, but the pain is never so severe as to cause vomiting. The cornea remains bright and the pupil tends to go into spasm and is smaller than on the normal side (Figure 7.3). Acute iritis is seen from time to time mainly in the 20–40-year age group, whereas acute glaucoma is extremely rare at these ages. Unless severe and bilateral, acute iritis is

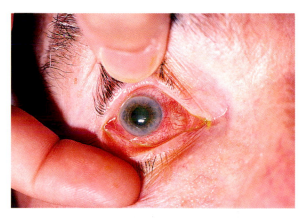

Fig. 7.2. Acute angle closure glaucoma.

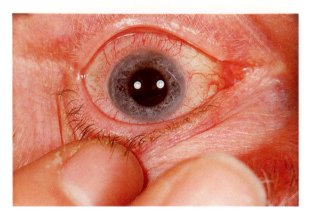

Fig. 7.3. Acute iritis. The pupil has been dilated with drops.

treated on an outpatient basis with local steroids and mydriatic drops. Some expertise is needed in the use of the correct mydriatic, and systemic steroids should be avoided unless the sight is in jeopardy. Because the iris forms part of the uvea, acute iritis is the same as acute anterior uveitis. In many cases no systemic cause can be found but it is important to exclude the possibility of sarcoidosis or ankylosing spondylitis. The condition lasts for about two weeks but tends to recur over a period of years. After two or three recurrences there is a high risk of the development of cataract, although this may form slowly.

Acute Keratitis

The characteristic features are sharp pain, often described as a foreign body in the eye, marked watering of the eye, photophobia and difficulty in opening the affected eye. The clinical picture is very different from those of the above two conditions and the commonest causes are the herpes simplex virus or trauma. The possibility of a perforating injury must always be borne in mind. Sometimes children are reticent about any history of injury for fear of incriminating a friend, and sometimes a small perforating injury is surprisingly painless. The treatment of acute keratitis has already been discussed in Chapter 6 and the management of corneal injuries will be considered in Chapter 16.

Thrombotic Glaucoma

The elderly patient who presents with a blind and painful eye and who may also be diabetic should be suspected of having thrombotic glaucoma. A fairly well-defined sequence of events enables the diagnosis to be inferred from the history. The first event is occlusion of the central retinal vein on one side and the patient notices that the vision of one eye has become blurred. Some elderly patients do not seek attention at this stage and some degree of spontaneous recovery may seem to occur before the onset of secondary glaucoma. Fortunately, only a modest proportion of cases develops this severe complication, which usually occurs, surprisingly enough, after 100 days, hence the term "a hundred-day glaucoma". Once the intraocular pressure rises, the eye tends to become painful and eventually degenerates in the absence of treatment, and sometimes even in spite of treatment. Thrombotic glaucoma remains as one of the few indications for surgical removal of the eye.

Failing Vision 8

Failing vision means that the sight as measured by the standard test type is worsening. The patient may say "I can't see so well doctor" or they may feel that their spectacles need changing. Some patients may not notice visual loss especially if it is in one eye. Sometimes more specific symptoms are given; the vision may be blurred, for example, in a patient with cataract, or objects may appear distorted or straight lines bent if there is disease of the macular region of the retina. Disease of the macular may also make objects look larger or smaller. Double vision is an important symptom since it can be the result of a cranial nerve palsy but if monocular it may be due to cataract. Patients quite often complain of floating black spots. If these move slowly with eye movement they may be due to some disturbance of the vitreous gel in the centre of the eye. If they are accompanied by seeing flashing lights the possibility of damage to the retina needs to be kept in mind. "Vitreous floaters" are very common and in most instances are of little pathological significance. Patients quite often notice haloes around lights and although this is typical of an attack of acute glaucoma haloes are also seen by patients with cataracts. Like many such symptoms they are best not asked for specifically. The question "do you ever see haloes?" is likely to be followed by the answer "yes". Night blindness is another such symptom. No one can see too well in the dark but if a patient has noticed a definite worsening of his or her ability to see in dim light, then an inherited retinal degeneration such as retinitis pigmentosa may be the cause.

Failing Vision in an Eye Which Looks Normal

When the Fundus is Normal

Very often a patient will present with a reduction of vision in one or both eyes and yet the eyes themselves look outwardly quite normal. In the case of a child, the parents may have noticed an apparent difficulty in reading or the vision may have been noticed to be poor at a routine school eye test. The next step is to decide whether the fundus is also normal but before dilating the pupil to allow fundus examination it is important to check the pupil reactions and to eliminate the possibility of refractive error. Once the glasses have been checked and the fundus examined then the presence of a normal fundus narrows the field down considerably. The likely diagnosis depends on the age of the patient. Infants with visual deterioration may require an examination under anaesthesia to exclude the possibility of a rare inherited retinal degeneration or other retinal disease. Other children, particularly those in the age group from nine to 12 years, must first be suspected of some emotional upset, perhaps due to domestic upheaval or stress at school. This may make them reluctant to read the test type. Sometimes such children discover that exercising their own power of accommodation produces blurring of vision and they may present with accommodation spasm.

The commonest cause of unilateral visual loss in children is amblyopia of disuse. This important cause of visual loss with a normal fundus is considered in more detail in the chapter on squint (Chapter 14). When, for any reason, one retina fails to receive a clear and correctly orientated image for a period of months or years during the time of visual development, then the sight of the eye remains impaired. The condition is treatable if caught before the visual reflexes are fully developed, that is, before the age of eight years. Young adults who present with unilateral visual loss and normal fundi may, of course, have amblyopia of disuse and the condition may be confirmed by looking for a squint or a refractive error more marked on the affected side.

We must also remember that retrobulbar neuritis presents in young people as sudden loss of vision on one side with aching behind the eye and a reduced pupil reaction on the affected side. This contrasts with amblyopia of disuse in which the pupil is normal. Migraine is another possibility to be considered in such patients.

Elderly patients who present with visual loss and normal fundi may give the history of a stroke and are found to have a homonymous hemianopic defect of the visual fields due to an embolus or thrombosis in the area of distribution of the posterior cerebral artery. Hysteria and malingering are also causes of unexplained visual loss, but these are extremely rare and it is important that the patient is investigated very carefully before such a diagnosis is made.

When the Fundus is Abnormal

Quite a proportion of patients who complain of loss of vision with eyes that look normal on superficial inspection show changes on ophthalmoscopy. The three important potentially blinding but eminently treatable ophthalmological conditions must be born in mind: cataract, chronic glaucoma and retinal detachment. It is an unfortunate fact that the commonest cause of visual loss in the elderly is usually untreatable at the present time. It is known as age-related macular degeneration and forms part of the sensory deprivation, which is an increasing scourge in elderly people. These diseases are limited to the eye itself, but disease elsewhere in the body can often first present as a visual problem. In this context we must remember what has been the commonest cause of blindness in young people – diabetic retinopathy, as well as the occasional case of severe hypertension. Intracranial causes of visual loss are perhaps less common in general practice and for this reason are easily missed. Intracranial tumours may present in an insidious manner, in particular the pituitary adenoma, and the diagnosis may be first suspected by careful plotting of the visual fields. In the case of the elderly patient who complains of visual deterioration in one eye, the ophthalmoscope all too commonly reveals age-related macular degeneration but it is also common to find that the patient has suffered a thrombosis of the central retinal vein or one of its branches. Unlike the situation with a central retinal artery occlusion, which is less common, some vision is preserved with a central retinal vein thrombosis in spite of the dramatic haemorrhagic fundus appearance. Temporal arteritis is another important vascular cause of visual failure in the elderly.

Finally, there are a large number of less common conditions, only one or two of which will be mentioned at this point. At any age the ingestion of drugs may affect the eyesight but there are very few proven oculotoxic drugs still on the market. One important example is chloroquine. When a dose of 100 g in one year is exceeded there is a risk of retinotoxicity, which may not be reversible. Although age-related macular degeneration is normally seen in patients over 60 years, the same problem may occur in younger people often with a recognised inheritance pattern. A completely different condition may also affect the macular region of young adults known as central serous retinopathy. This tends to resolve spontaneously after a few weeks although treatment by laser coagulation is occasionally needed. Unilateral progressive visual loss in young people may also be due to posterior uveitis, which is the same thing as choroiditis. The known causes and management of this condition will be discussed in a later chapter (see chapter 18).

The more common causes of failing vision in a normal looking eye may be summarised as shown in Table 8.1.

Treatable Causes of Failing Vision

Nobody can deny that the practice of ophthalmology is highly effective. There are many eye diseases, which can be cured or arrested, and it is possible to restore the sight fully from total blindness. Many of the commoner causes of blindness especially in the third world are treatable. The most important treatable cause of visual failure in the UK is cataract, and

Table 8.1. Failing vision in a normal-looking eye

	Fundus Normal	**Fundus Abnormal**
Child	Refractive error Disuse amblyopia Inherited retinal degeneration Emotional stress	Cataract Macular degeneration Posterior uveitis
Young Adult	Refractive error Retrobulbar neuritis Intracranial space occupying lesion Drug toxicity	Diabetic retinopathy Retinal detachment Macular disease Hypertension Posterior uveitis
Elderly	Homonymous hemianopia	Macular degeneration Central vein thrombosis Chronic glaucoma Cataract Vitreous haemorrhage Temporal arteritis

of course no patient should be allowed to go blind from this cause although this does occasionally happen (Figure 8.1). Retinal detachment is less common than cataract but it provides a situation where the sight may be lost completely and then be fully restored. For the best results, surgery must be carried out as soon as possible, before the retina becomes degenerate, whereas delay prior to cataract surgery does not usually affect the outcome of the

operation. Acute glaucoma is another instance where the sight may be lost but restored by prompt treatment. The treatment of chronic glaucoma has less impression on the patient because it is aimed at preventing visual deterioration, although in sight saving terms it may be equally effective.

It is very easy to overlook the value of antibiotics in saving sight. Prior to their introduction, many more eyes had to be removed following injury and infection. Systemic and locally applied steroids also play a sight-saving role in the management of temporal arteritis in the elderly and in the treatment of uveitis. In recent years the treatment of diabetic retinopathy has been greatly advanced by the combined effect of laser coagulation and scrupulous control of the diabetes. In the past, about one-half of the of the patients with the proliferative type of retinopathy would be expected to go blind over five years and many of these were young people at the height of their careers. The proper management of ocular trauma often has a great influence on the visual result, and the rare but dreaded complication of ocular perforating injuries – sympathetic ophthalmia – can now be effectively treated with systemic steroids. Amblyopia of disuse has already been mentioned; the treatment is undoubtedly effective in some cases but the results are disappointing if the diagnosis is made when the child is too old or when there is poor patient co-operation.

Untreatable Causes of Failing Vision

Ophthalmologists are sometimes asked if the sight can be restored to a blind eye and, as a general rule, one can say that if there is no perception of light in the eye, then it is unlikely that the sight can be improved irrespective of the cause. There are several ophthalmological conditions for which there is no known effective treatment and it is sometimes important that the patient is made aware of this at an early stage in order to avoid unnecessary anxiety, and perhaps unnecessary visits to the doctor. Most degenerative diseases of the retina fail to respond to treatment. If the retina is out of place, it can be replaced, but old retinae cannot be replaced with new. So far there has been no firm evidence that any drug can alter the course of inherited retinal degenerations such as retinitis pigmentosa, although useful information is beginning to appear about the biochemistry and genetics of these conditions.

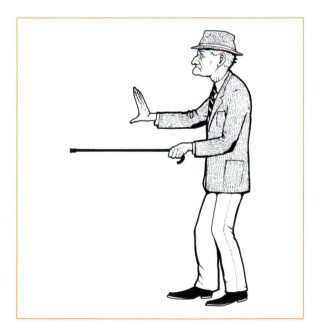

Fig. 8.1. The family thought it was just old age.

Age-related macular degeneration tends to run a progressive course in spite of any attempts at treatment, and although most patients do not become completely blind, it accounts for loss of reading vision in many elderly people. Some myopic patients are susceptible to degeneration of the retina in later years; known as myopic chorioretinal degeneration, it may account for visual deterioration in myopes who have otherwise undergone successful cataract or retinal surgery.

Scarring of the retina following trauma is another cause of permanent and untreatable visual loss, but the most dramatic and irrevocable loss of vision occurs following traumatic section of the optic nerve. One must be careful here before dismissing the patient as untreatable because on rare occasions a contusion injury to the eye or orbit may result in a haemorrhage into the sheath of the optic nerve. Some degree of visual recovery may sometimes occur in these patients and it has been claimed that recovery may be helped by surgically opening the nerve sheath. There is one odd exception to this dramatic form of blindness which may follow optic nerve insult; visual loss due to optic neuritis. Patients with retrobulbar neuritis (optic neuritis) nearly always recover their vision again whether they receive treatment or not. The explanation is that the visual loss is due to pressure from oedema rather than to damage to the nerve fibres themselves. It is hardly necessary to say that any neurological damage proximal to the optic nerve tends to produce permanent and untreatable visual loss, as exemplified by the homonymous hemianopic field defect which may follow a cerebrovascular accident.

Malignant tumours of the eye come into this category of untreatable causes of visual failure but in fact serious attempts are now being made to treat them with radiotherapy in specialised units and the prognosis appears to be improving in some cases.

Headache 9

Headache must be one of the commonest symptoms, and few specialties escape from the diagnostic problems that it may present. We must begin with the realisation that more or less everyone suffers from headache at some time or other. In fact, the majority of headaches that present have no detectable cause and are often labelled psychogenic if there seems to be a background of stress. The implication is that the sufferer is perhaps exaggerating mild symptoms in order to gain sympathy from his or her spouse, or even perhaps the doctor. One must, of course, be extremely cautious about not accepting symptoms at their face value, and certainly cerebral tumours have been overlooked for this very reason. If the psychogenic headache is the commonest, then the headache due to raised intracranial pressure and a space-occupying lesion must be the most important. Between these two the whole spectrum of causes must be considered. It is essential, therefore, to memorise a permanent checklist in order that obvious causes are not omitted.

History

Often the history is the total disease in the absence of any physical signs and it is important to note the nature of the pain, the total duration and frequency of the pain, the time of day it occurs, and its relation to other events or the taking of analgesics. Headaches that are present "all the time" and are described in fanciful terms tend not to have an organic basis; the patient with an organic headache is not usually smiling. The time of day may be important: raised intracranial pressure has the reputation of causing an early morning headache which is described as bursting or throbbing and which may be made worse by straining or coughing. We must always remember the triad of headache, vomiting and papilloedema in this respect, especially as the vomiting may not be accompanied by nausea, and is not necessarily mentioned by the patient. The family history should also be noted especially where there is a history of migraine.

Classification

When considering the different common causes of headache, an anatomical classification is a useful way of providing a reference list. The following should be considered by the examining doctor.

Cerebrospinal Fluid

A rise or fall from normal of the cerebrospinal fluid pressure is associated with headache. When the cerebrospinal fluid pressure is raised the patient usually experiences a bursting pain, which may interrupt sleep or appear in the early morning. It tends to be intermittent and made worse by coughing or lying down. It may also, of course, be accompanied by papilloedema and vomiting, and another important symptom is blurring and transient obscurations of vision. The situation of the pain is usually diffuse rather focal, but we must remember that a bursting headache made worse by coughing is sometimes described by otherwise healthy individuals. When the rise of intracranial pressure is due to a space-occupying lesion, signs of focal brain damage may also be present.

63

Blood Vessels

A variety of diseases involving the blood vessels may cause headache. The commonest is probably migraine. Classical migraine is thought to be due to an initial spasm followed by dilatation of the meningeal arteries. There is usually a family history of the same problem showing dominant inheritance, and attacks may sometimes be precipitated by stress or taking certain foods such as cheese. Before the headache begins there is usually a visual aura characterised by a shimmering effect before one or both eyes which spreads across the vision, or the appearance of zig-zag lines known as fortifications because of their resemblance to the silhouette of a fortress. The visual disturbance may take the form of a hemianopic scotoma or, very rarely, of a formed hallucination but, whatever their nature, they tend to last for about 10–20 min and are followed by a headache which is centred above eye and is described as a boring pain. The headache lasts for anytime between 1 and 24 h and then disperses. The patient may experience nausea and vomiting as the attack ends. Migraine may begin quite early in childhood and continue at regular intervals for many years. Migraines are more common in women and tend to improve at the time of the menopause. Atypical migraine can sometimes pose a diagnostic problem. The visual aura may appear by itself or the migraine attack may be accompanied by gastrointestinal symptoms or by ophthalmoplegia. The attack may be preceded by oliguria and fluid retention and be followed by a diuresis. Very rarely, a permanent hemianopic scotoma or ophthalmoplegia may result from an attack of migraine, but in these circumstances the original diagnosis must be reviewed very carefully.

There is some doubt as to whether essential hypertension causes headaches but there is no doubt that when the blood pressure becomes acutely raised, a severe headache may ensue, accompanied by blurring of vision. Any adults with headaches should have their blood pressure measured. Another form of headache associated with abnormality of the blood vessels is that due to an intracranial aneurysm of the internal carotid artery or one of its branches. The pain in this case is usually throbbing in nature and there may be other signs of a space-occupying lesion at the apex of the orbit, for example, a cranial nerve palsy or a bruit heard with the stethoscope. In the case of elderly patients, the possibility of giant cell arteritis must always be kept in mind. This is an inflammation of the walls of

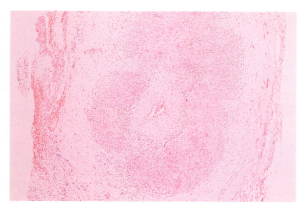

Fig. 9.1. Cross-section of the temporal artery from patient with temporal arteritis. The artery is almost occluded. Note the large number of giant cells (with acknowledgement to Dr J. Lowe).

many of the medium-sized arteries in the body but it tends to affect the temporal arteries preferentially. The walls of the vessels become thickened by inflammatory cells and giant cells mainly in the media and there is fibrosis of the intima (Figure 9.1). The lumen of the affected vessels becomes occluded. Affected patients are usually over the age of 70 years and complain of tenderness of the scalp, especially over the temporal arteries, which may be seen and felt to be inflamed, and no pulse can be felt in them. The headache is made particularly bad by attempting to brush the hair and other symptoms include jaw claudication. The importance of this type of headache rests on the fact that the eye is involved in about 60% of cases and the patient may suddenly go blind in one eye and then a short time later blind in the other. The diagnosis depends on finding a markedly raised erythroctye sedimentation rate (ESR) (above 70 mm/h) and if necessary performing a temporal artery biopsy. Whenever an elderly patient presents with occlusive vascular disease in the eye and a high ESR, this diagnosis should be considered because it is possible to treat the condition by means of systemic steroids. In practice, it is the ciliary arteries that become occluded and the central retinal artery is involved in only about 5% of cases. Once steroids have been instituted, the dose should be very carefully monitored, preferably in co-operation with a general physician, with regular measurement of the ESR. Other less common vascular causes of headache include intracranial angioma and subarachnoid or subdural haemorrhage.

Blood

Changes in the blood itself may also be associated with headache. It is easy to forget that anaemic patients often have headaches, which can be cured by treating the anaemia. Likewise, patients with polycythaemia may also complain of headache. Hypoglycaemia is another recognised cause; here the symptoms occur after strenuous exercise or insulin excess in a diabetic patient.

Nerves

Cluster headache. In many respects this type of headache resembles migraine although it is more common in men in the third or fourth decade. The word "cluster" refers to the timing of the attacks, which may be repeated several times over a few weeks followed by a period of remission for several months. The pain is described as being very severe and unilateral. There is conjunctival congestion and constriction of the pupil on the affected side, and the attack may last from minutes to hours. Tenderness over the side of the face and nasal discharge are also features. Raeder's paratrigeminal neuralgia probably merges with cluster headache, being described as severe ocular pain associated with meiosis and ptosis. Trigeminal neuralgia can be easily distinguished from these other forms of headache by its distribution over one or all of the terminal branches of the trigeminal nerve and the fact that the very severe pain is triggered by touching a part of the cheek or by chewing and swallowing. The pain is so severe that the patient may become suicidal, and surgical division of the trigeminal nerve at the level of the Gasserian ganglion has been a method of treatment.

Post-herpetic neuralgia is an extremely debilitating form of headache experienced by elderly people after an attack of trigeminal herpes zoster. The pain seems to be more severe in the elderly and it may persist for many years. The cause of the headache is usually evident when one inspects the skin of the forehead, which is slightly whitened and scarred from the previous attack of herpes zoster. Apart from the use of analgesics, antidepressant drugs may also help, together with the application of local heat or vibration massage. Fortunately the prompt treatment of the original attack of herpes zoster at primary care level with systemic acyclovir does seem to be reducing the incidence of this troublesome condition.

Bones

Paget's disease of bone. In this condition the bones of the head enlarge and grow abnormally, the abnormal growth being associated with headache and incidentally an increase in hat size. The eyes themselves may show optic atrophy, and close inspection of the fundi may reveal the curious appearance of wavy lines known as angioid streaks. Oxycephaly is a congenital defect of the skull due to premature closure of the sutures; patients sometimes complain of headache as well as visual loss due to optic nerve compression. Multiple myeloma is the name given to a malignant proliferation of plasma cells within the bone marrow. There is also an excessive production of immunoglobulins. Osteolytic bone lesions occur especially in the skull, and headache may be an accompaniment. The disease is more common in the elderly and is accompanied by a high ESR. Diagnosis is made by examining the urine for Bence-Jones protein and the serum for abnormal immunoglobulins. Disease of the cervical vertebrae is another cause of headache, due to the effect of spasm of the neck muscles. Relief of the pain by neck manipulation has been claimed but the exact diagnosis must be made before embarking on such treatment.

Meninges

It is presumed that the pain and headache, which accompany meningitis or encephalitis, are mediated through the sensory nerve supply to the meninges. The pain sensitive structures in the middle and anterior cranial fossa are supplied by the Vth cranial nerve, and inflammation may produce referred pain to the region of the eye.

The Eyes

The classical eye headache is that of subacute narrow angle glaucoma. Here the headache is an evening one, tends to be over one eye and is nearly always accompanied by blurring of vision and seeing coloured haloes around street lights. If the intraocular pressure is measured when the headache is present and is found to be normal, then it is unlikely that narrow angle glaucoma is the correct diagnosis. On the other hand, the diagnosis cannot be so easily excluded if the headache is absent at the time of examination. Patients with narrow angle glaucoma are long sighted – therefore beware the middle-aged long-sighted patient with evening headaches and blurring of vision. Chronic open angle glaucoma very rarely causes headache because the rise of intraocular pressure is too gradual and not great enough. The possibility should be borne in mind when a patient experiences headaches following ocular trauma or eye surgery, that there may be secondary glaucoma. This type of glaucoma often responds well to treatment but if ignored may lead rapidly to blindness. Acute iritis is associated with headache but in practice rarely presents as such because the other ocular symptoms override this. Patients developing endophthalmitis complain of severe pain in the eye and headache, this being a particularly important symptom following cataract surgery.

It has been argued that refractive error does not cause headache, but nothing could be further from the truth. Refractive headache is most commonly seen in uncorrected hypermetropes, sometimes in children, but more commonly in adults aged 30–40 years who are beginning to have difficulty in accommodating through their long sightedness. For reasons of vanity, patients may have been deliberately avoiding the use of glasses and it may have to be explained to them that they have the choice of having headaches or wearing glasses. In the patient with no refractive error, the onset of presbyopia may be accompanied by headache, which is sometimes delayed until the morning after prolonged reading. An otherwise normal person aged 45 years should be suspected of having presbyopic headaches. Uncorrected myopes do not usually complain of headaches. If the spectacle prescription is incorrect for any reason then a sensitive person may experience headache, but it is surprising how some people will tolerate an incorrect spectacle lens without complaint. Ocular muscle imbalance is an uncommon cause of headache but it is an important one because it can be corrected with considerable relief to the patient. Usually the patient shows a considerable difference in refractive error between the two eyes and when the eyes are dissociated by such means as the cover test or the Maddox wing test, one eye tends to drift upwards or downwards. Relief of symptoms may be achieved by incorporating a prism into the spectacle lens or, if the deviation is marked by ocular muscle surgery. Horizontal imbalance of the ocular movements is less closely linked with headache, although there is a group of patients, usually young adults under stress, who seem unable to converge their eyes on near objects; instead they allow one eye to drift outwards when reading. Some elderly patients have the same problem but do not so often have associated headache. This so-called convergence insufficiency can be greatly improved by a course of convergence exercises and provides one of the few instances where exercises of the eye muscles have any therapeutic value.

Pain Referred from Other Sites

Sinusitis is well recognised as a common cause of headache and the patient with headache should be questioned about recent upper respiratory tract infections or a previous history of sinus disease. Tenderness over the affected sinus is an important sign. The headache tends to begin after rising in the morning and reaches a peak later in the morning. Pain from an infected tooth may be referred over the side of the face and cause some diagnostic confusion but it is usually worse when chewing or biting. Pain from a middle ear infection may cause similar problems. The temporomandibular joint is a recognised source of referred pain over the side of the face, and malfunctioning of the joint may result from incorrect jaw alignment or poorly fitting dentures.

Drugs

Over-indulgence in alcohol is one of the three causes of morning headache; the other two being raised intracranial pressure and acute sinusitis. The diagnostic difficulty with alcoholism tends to be failure of the patient to admit or recognise excessive drinking. It may seem strange that such a patient should ever seek a doctor's opinion about headache, but alcoholics do sometimes seek an ophthalmological opinion for their symptoms without relating them to alcohol intake and perhaps urged on by an anxious relative or friend. Chronic poisoning by other drugs is too rare a cause of headache in ophthalmic practice to be considered here but it may have to be kept in mind.

Post-traumatic Headache

Nearly all patients who have suffered a significant head injury complain of headaches. The pain may remain severe for many months and in the worst case may last a few years. Usually no obvious explanation can be found apart from the original injury. The severity of the headache may sometimes appear to be related to clinical depression following the injury but other causes of headache such as ocular muscle imbalance or raised intracranial pressure need to be excluded.

Contact Lenses 10

The widespread use of contact lenses means that the general practitioner and the ophthalmic casualty department find themselves confronted with more and more patients who have run into wearing problems of one kind or another. For this reason some of the likely emergency requirements are considered here.

Types

As long ago as 1912 a glass contact lens was being produced, but because of the manufacturing difficulties and wearing problems, the widespread use of this type of optical aid was delayed until the introduction of plastic scleral lenses in 1937. "Hard" lenses are made from the non-toxic plastic material of Perspex or polymethylmethacrylate (PMMA). The obvious advantage of placing a lens directly on the cornea over the wearing of spectacles is the cosmetic one, but the system also has optical advantages. Because the lens moves with the eye there are none of the problems associated with looking through the edge of the lens experienced by the wearer of spectacles. In addition, a more subtle effect is the more accurate representation of image size on the retina in subjects with high degrees of refractive error.

Although the moulded scleral contact lenses are still occasionally used, they have been largely replaced by the modern "hard lens" which is much smaller and thinner and hence causes less interference with corneal physiology. In 1960 the hydrophilic contact lens was introduced. This had the great advantage of being soft and malleable and hence more comfortable to wear, but optically it has never been quite as good as the hard lens, especially when the patient has high degrees of astigmatism.

Several different materials have now been used in the production of soft lenses although the basic material used is hydroxmethylmethacrylate (HEMA). The different types of soft lenses differ in their ability to take up water or oxygen. Lenses are now being made which can be worn for long periods without needing to be removed and cleaned. Similarly, disposable contact lenses are now widely available. Care should be taken that such lenses are used under professional care.

Soft contact lenses tend to absorb and adsorb material from the tear film. It is particularly important to ensure that a patient is not wearing a soft lens before fluorescein dye is instilled into the eye.

Gas-permeable lenses are made from a mixture of hard and soft lens material. They combine the ease of wear of soft lenses with reduced side-effects (especially long-term) of hard lenses.

Side-effects

In general, soft contact lenses have more side-effects than hard lenses in the long term. The commonest complication of wearing modern contact lenses is losing them. Patients are well advised to have a pair of glasses at hand in case they have contact-lens-wearing problems or a lens is lost. More serious trouble may result from clumsy handling of the lens or leaving a hard lens in the eye for too long a period. Such patients quite often present with severe pain in the eye, and examination reveals a partially healed corneal abrasion. This must be treated in the usual manner and the patient advised against wearing the lens again for several weeks, depending on the extent of the abrasion. The contact lenses themselves should also be examined by the patient's fitter to make sure that they are not faulty. Bearing in mind the troubles, which may ensue when an abrasion becomes recurrent, the indications for wearing the lenses in the first place should be reconsidered.

The risk of infections by lens contamination or secondary to corneal abrasions is increased. Recently acanthamoeba keratitis has been described. This disease occurs more often in contact lens wearers.

Another sequel to wearing contact lenses, either hard or soft, is the appearance of chronic inflammatory changes in the conjunctiva, often characterised by a papillary conjunctivitis. The resulting irritation and redness of the eyes may persist for some weeks after the wearing of the contact lenses ceases. Unfortunately these symptoms may appear after wearing lenses successfully for some years and they may tend to recur in spite of renewing the lenses. Some patients who tolerate contact lenses very well may develop corneal changes after some years. Peripheral vascularisation may become evident and in neglected cases there may be band degeneration of the cornea. Some contact-lens wearers complain of recurrent blurring of their vision and this may be due to an ill-fitting lens producing corneal epithelial oedema or simply to the excessive accumulation of mucus on the lens (Figure 10.1).

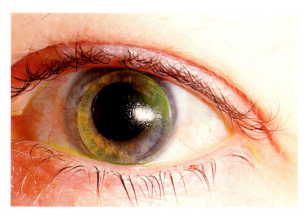

Fig. 10.1. Hard contact lens with lipid deposits (with acknowledgement to Professor M. Rubinstein).

Indications

These may be considered as either cosmetic or therapeutic.

Cosmetic

There are obvious cosmetic advantages for the wearer of contact lenses, especially the teenager. However, the potential wearer should realise the possible difficulties involved: the need to clean and sterilise the lenses and the need for some degree of finger dexterity when they are inserted and removed. They may be required for certain pursuits such as golf or athletics where the spectacle wearer is handicapped by misting up of the glasses in wet weather. Patients over the age of 45 or 50 years will find that they require reading glasses as well and these, of course, must be worn over the contact lenses, thereby somewhat reducing the cosmetic value of the latter.

Therapeutic

There are instances when the contact lens may result in much better vision than spectacles, for example in patients with high degrees of corneal astigmatism which are not fully correctable with glasses. This accounts for the benefit of contact lenses in patients with keratoconus. Soft contact lenses are sometimes used as "bandage lenses" to protect the cornea after corneal burns or in patients with bullous keratopathy. The contact lens has a special importance in the correction of unilateral aphakia (see Chapter 11) by reducing the image size on the retina to such an extent that the two eyes can once again be used together. If eye drops are being regularly instilled into the eyes, soft contact lenses may absorb the drug being used or the preservative in the drops. In fact, attempts have been made to use soft contact lenses as a slow-release system by impregnating them with the drug before fitting.

Section III

Problems of the Eye Surgeon

The eye surgeon is confronted by problems, which have been selected to a greater or lesser extent by the general practitioner or the optometrist. In the larger teaching centres he or she may be in a position to see patients selected in turn by other ophthalmologists and thus may be able to gain a very detailed experience of relatively few aspects of the subject. In this section the cardinal eye problems which confront any eye surgeon are described. Being surgical problems, they are all fairly rapidly responsive to treatment, sometimes involving the restoration of sight to the blind patient. In other cases the surgical treatment may simply arrest or delay the progress of visual failure or relieve the patient of pain or discomfort.

"Cataract" means an opacity of the lens, and it is the commonest potentially blinding condition which confronts the eye surgeon. This is not to say that every person with cataract is liable to go blind. Many patients have relatively slight lens opacities that progress very slowly. Fortunately the results of surgery are very good, a satisfactory improvement of vision being obtained in about 90% of cases. It is usually possible to forewarn the patients when there is an additional element of doubt about the outcome. To the uninformed patient "cataract" strikes a note of fear and it may be necessary to explain that opacities in the lens are extremely common in elderly people. It is only when the opaque lens fibres begin to interfere with the vision that the term "cataract" is used. Many patients have a slight degree of cataract, which advances so slowly that they die before any visual problems arise. Nobody need now go blind from cataract; however one still encounters elderly people who from ignorance or neglect, are left immobilised by this form of blindness, and it is especially important that the general practitioner is able to recognise the condition.

The Lens

The human lens is a surprising structure. It is avascular and yet it is actively growing throughout life, albeit extremely slowly. It receives its nourishment from the aqueous fluid that bathes it. The lens is enclosed in an elastic capsule and for this reason tends to assume a spherical shape, or would do if the moulding of the lens fibres allowed.

In situ the shape of the lens is maintained by a series of taut fibres known as the zonule. The fibres exert radial tension on the lens but the tension is reduced when the circular part of the ciliary muscle contracts. The reduced tension of the zonule allows the lens to assume a more spherical shape and hence the anteroposterior diameter of the lens increases. As a result, the refracting power of the lens increases, that is to say, light rays are more bent and the eye becomes focused on near objects. This process of accommodation, which is produced by relaxation of the lens but contraction of the ciliary muscle, gradually becomes less effective as we grow older, probably because the lens becomes less malleable rather than because the ciliary muscle is becoming weaker. This reduction in the range of accommodation explains why the small child will present an object close to an adult's eyes and expect him or her to see it clearly. It also explains why, in the mid-40s it becomes necessary to hold a book further from ones eyes if it is to be read easily and also the subsequent inability to read without the assistance of a spectacle lens which provides additional converging power. The need for reading glasses occurs in people with normal eyes at about the age of 45 years (presbyopia), but this is only a milestone in a slowly progressive path of deterioration that begins at birth.

Histological section of the lens reveals that beneath the capsule there is an anterior epithelium with a single layer of cells, but no such layer is evident beneath the posterior capsule. Furthermore, if one follows the single-layered anterior epithelium to the equator of the lens, then the epithelial cells can be seen to elongate progressively and lose their nuclei as they are traced into the interior of the lens. Thus one can deduce from histological sections that the lens fibres are being continuously laid down from the epithelial cells at the equator. The actual arrangement of the lens fibres is quite complex;

each fibre being made up of a prismatic six-sided band bound to its fellow by an amorphous cement substance.

Slit-lamp examination of the lens reveals the presence of the lens sutures, which mark the points of junction of the end of the lens fibres. Two such sutures are usually seen, both often taking the form of the letter "Y", the posterior suture being inverted. The lens fibres contain proteins known as "crystallins" and have the property of setting up an antigen-antibody reaction if they are released into the eye from the lens capsule. One other feature of the lens which can usually be seen with slit-lamp microscope is an object looking like a pig's tail which hangs from the posterior capsule. This is the remains of the hyaloid artery, a vessel that runs in the embryonic eye from the optic disc to the vascular tunic of the lens, which is present at that stage (Figure 11.1).

Aetiology

Having learned of the complex structure of the lens, perhaps one should be more surprised that the lens retains its transparency throughout life than that some of the lens fibres may become opaque. There are a number of reasons why lens fibres become opaque but the commonest and most important is ageing. The various causes will now be considered.

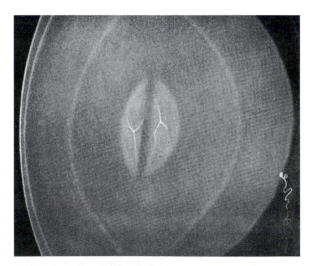

Fig. 11.1. Cross-section of a child's lens: aqueous on left, vitreous on right. Note the hyaloid remnant and the "Y" sutures (with acknowledgement to M. L. Berliner, 1949).

Age

The majority of cataracts are associated with the ageing process, and some of the biochemical changes in the lens fibres are now being understood. We know that certain families are more susceptible to age-related cataract, but a degree of opacification of the lens is commonplace in the elderly. Often the opacity is limited to the peripheral part of the lens and the patient may be unaware of any problem. It is usual to limit the term "cataract" to the situation where the opacities are causing some degree of visual impairment. Elderly patients are often reassured to learn that their eye condition is part of the general ageing process and that only in certain instances does the opacification progress to the point where surgery is required.

Diabetes

The new house surgeon working in an eye ward must be impressed by the number of diabetics with cataracts who pass through his or her hands, and might be forgiven for deducing that diabetes is a common cause of cataract. To see the situation in perspective one must realise that both cataracts and diabetes are common diseases of the elderly and coincide quite often. Of course, the matter has been investigated from the statistical point of view and it has been shown that there is a somewhat higher incidence of cataract in diabetics, mainly because they tend to develop lens opacities at an earlier age. A special type of cataract is seen in young diabetics and in these cases the lens may become rapidly opaque in a few months. Fortunately this is not very common, usually occurring in insulin-dependent patients who have had difficulty with the control of their diabetes. It is claimed that in its early stages this type of cataract can be reversible, but such an occurrence is so rare that it has not presented much opportunity for study.

Secondary

Cataract may be secondary to disease in the eye or disease elsewhere in the body.

Secondary to Disease in the Eye

More or less any terminal event in the eye tends to be associated with cataract. Advanced uncontrolled glaucoma is often associated with an opaque lens, as are chronic iridocyclitis and intraocular tumours.

Certain specific eye diseases are accompanied by cataract; for example, patients who suffer from the inherited retinal degeneration, retinitis pigmentosa, sometimes develop a particular type of opacity in the posterior part of the lens. The removal of such a cataract may sometimes restore a considerable amount of vision, at least for a time.

Secondary to Disease Elsewhere

It may be recalled that the lens is ectodermal, being developed as an invagination of the overlying surface ectoderm. It is not surprising therefore, that some skin diseases are associated with cataract. In particular patients suffering from asthma and eczema may present to the eye surgeon in their late 50s. Dysfunction of the parathyroid glands is a very rare cause of cataract and Down's syndrome is a more common association.

Trauma

Contusion

A direct blow on the eye, if it is severe enough, may cause the lens to become opaque. A squash-ball injury is a typical example of the type of force required. Sometimes the appearance of the cataract may be delayed even for several years. The onset of unilateral cataract must always make one suspect the possibility of previous injury, but a cause-and-effect relationship may be difficult to prove in the absence of any other signs of previous contusion. It seems unlikely that a cataract would form unless there had been a direct blow on the eye itself, although occasionally medicolegal claims are made for compensation when a cataract has developed following a blow on the side of the head.

Perforation

A perforating wound of the eye bears a much higher risk of cataract formation. If the perforating object (for example, a broken beer glass) passes through the cornea without touching the lens, then usually the lens is spared and, in the absence of significant contusion, a cataract does not form. This, of course, also depends on careful management of the corneal wound and the prevention of infection. Unfortunately such perforating injuries may also involve splitting of the lens capsule with spilling out of the lens fibres into the anterior chamber. The series of events, which follow such an injury, is dependent on the age of the individual. When the lens capsule of a child is ruptured, a vigorous inflammatory reaction is set up in the anterior chamber and the lens matter will usually gradually become absorbed, in the absence of treatment, over a period of about a month. This leaves behind the lens capsule and often a clear pupil. In spite of this the patient cannot see clearly because most of the refractive power of the eye is lost. This has serious optical consequences and the need for an artificial intraocular lens. When the lens capsule of an adult is ruptured, a similar inflammatory reaction ensues, but there tends to be more fibrosis, and a white plaque of fibrous tissue may remain to obstruct the pupil. Very rarely, it is possible for a lens to be perforated with subsequent opacity limited to the site of perforation – indeed, one occasionally sees a foreign body within the lens surrounded by opaque fibres but limited to a small part of the lens.

Radiation

Visible light does not seem to cause cataract, although claims have been made that individuals from white races living for long periods in the tropics may show a higher incidence of cataract. In practice this is not easy to confirm. In spite of public misapprehension, ultraviolet light probably does not cause cataract either, since the shorter wavelengths fail to penetrate the globe. These shorter wavelengths beyond the blue end of the visible spectrum can produce a dramatic superficial burn of the cornea, which usually heals in about 48 h. This injury, which is typified by "snow blindness" and "welder's flash", will be discussed in Chapter 15. Prolonged doses of infrared rays can produce cataract; this used to seen occasionally in glass-blowers and steel workers, but the wearing of goggles has now more or less eliminated this. X-rays and g-rays may also produce cataracts, as was witnessed by the mass of reports, which followed the explosion of the atomic bombs at Nagasaki and Hiroshima. Radiation cataract is now seen following whole-body radiation for leukaemia but the risk is only significant when therapeutic doses of X-rays are used.

Congenital Factors

Many of the cases of congenital cataract seen in ophthalmic practice are inherited. Sometimes there is a dominant family history and there are many other possible associated defects, some of which fit into named syndromes. Acquired congenital cataract may result from maternal rubella infection during the first trimester of pregnancy. The association of deafness, congenital heart lesions and cataract must always be born in mind. The ophthalmic house surgeon must take special care when examining the congenital cataract case preoperatively and likewise the paediatric house surgeon must bear in mind that congenital cataracts may be overlooked, especially if they are not very severe. Sometimes the cataracts may be slight at birth and gradually progress subsequently, or sometimes they may remain stationary until later years.

Toxicity

Toxic cataracts are probably rare, although several currently used drugs have been incriminated, the most notable being systemic steroids. Chlorpromazine has also been shown to cause lens opacities in large doses, and so has the use of certain miotics, including pilocarpine. Much of our knowledge of drug-induced cataracts is based on former animal experiments. The potential danger of new drugs causing cataract was shown in the 1930s after the introduction of dinitrophenol as a slimming agent. This produced a large number of lens opacities before it was eventually withdrawn.

Symptoms

Many patients complain of blurred vision, which is usually worse when viewing distant objects. If the patient is unable to read small print, the surgeon may suspect that other pathology such as macular degeneration may be present. One must bear in mind that some elderly patients say that they cannot read when it is found that they *can* read small print when carefully tested. It is a curious fact that when the cataract is unilateral the patient may claim that the loss of vision has been quite sudden. Elucidation of the history in these cases sometimes reveals that the visual loss was noted when washing and observing the face in the mirror. When one hand is lowered before the other, the unilateral visual loss is noticed for the first time and interpreted as a sudden event. The history in cataract cases may be further confused by a natural tendency for patients to project their symptoms into the spectacles, and several pairs may be obtained before the true cause of the problem is found.

In order to understand the symptoms of cataract it is essential to understand what is meant by index myopia. This simply refers to the change in refractive power of the lens, which occurs as a preliminary to cataract formation. Index myopia may also result from uncontrolled diabetes. If we imagine an elderly patient who requires reading glasses (for presbyopia) in the normal way but no glasses for viewing distant objects, then the onset of index myopia will produce blurring of distance vision, but also the patient will discover to his or her surprise that it is possible to read again without glasses. In the same way the hypermetropic patient will become less hypermetropic and find that it is possible to see again in the distance without glasses. The ageing fibres in the precataractous lens become more effective at converging light rays so that parallel rays of light are brought to a focus more anteriorly in the eye.

Apart from blurring of vision, the cataract patient often complains of monocular diplopia. Sometimes even a very slight and subtle opacity in the posterior part of the lens can cause the patient to notice, for example, that car rear lights appear doubled, and this may be reproduced with the ophthalmoscope light. Monocular diplopia is sometimes regarded as a rather suspect symptom, the suggestion being that if a patient continues to see double even when one eye is closed, then he or she may not be giving a very accurate history. In actual practice nothing could be further from the truth and this is quite a common presenting feature of cataract.

Glare is another common presenting symptom. The patient complains that he or she cannot see so well in bright light and may even be wearing a pair of dark glasses. Glare is a photographic term but here it refers to a significant reduction in visual acuity when an extraneous light source is introduced. Light shining from the side is scattered in the cataractous lens and reduces the quality of the image on the retina. Glare becomes an important consideration when advising an elderly cataractous patient on fitness to drive. The visual acuity may be within the requirements laid down by law (seeing a number plate at 67 ft or 20.5 m) but only when the patient is tested in the absence of glare.

A consideration of all these factors makes it relatively easy to diagnose cataract even before examining the patient. To summarise, a typical patient may complain that the glasses have been inaccurately prescribed, that the vision is much worse in bright sunlight, that sometimes things look double, and that there is difficulty in recognising peoples faces in the street rather than difficulty in reading. Patients with cataracts alone do not usually complain that things look distorted or that straight lines look bent, nor do they experience pain in the eye.

Very rarely, cataracts become hypermature; that is to say, the lens enlarges in the eye and this in turn may lead to secondary glaucoma and pain in the eye. Urgent surgery may be needed under these circumstances. In its late stages, a cataract matures and becomes white, so that exceptionally a patient may complain of a white spot in the middle of the pupil.

Signs

Reduced Visual Acuity

A reduction in visual acuity may, of course, be an early sign of cataract formation but this is not always the case. Some patients see surprisingly well through marked lens opacities, and the effect on visual acuity as measured by the Snellen test type depends as much on the position of the opacities in the lens as upon the density of the opacities.

Findings of Ophthalmoscopy

The best way of picking up a cataract in its early stages is to view the pupil through the ophthalmoscope from a distance of about 50 cm. In this way the red reflex is clearly seen. The red reflex is simply the reflection of light from the fundus and it is viewed in exactly the same manner that one might view cat's eyes in the headlamps of one's car or the eyes of one's friends in an ill-judged flash photograph. In fact such a flash photo could well show up an early

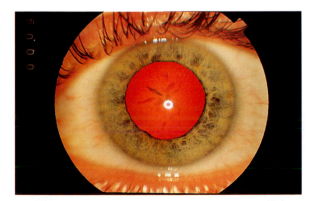

Fig. 11.2. Opaque areas in the lens can be seen clearly against the red reflex.

cataract if an elderly relative were included in the photograph. When using the ophthalmoscope, the opacities in the lens are often seen as black spokes against the red reflex (Figure 11.2). It is important to focus one's eyes on the plane of the patient's pupil if the cataract is to be well seen, and it is preferable to dilate the pupil beforehand or at least examine in a darkened room. Typical age-related lens opacities are wedge shaped, pointing towards the centre of the pupil. At the same time the central nucleus of the lens may take on a yellow–brown colour, the appearance being termed "lens sclerosis", and ultimately the lens may become nearly black in some instances.

After inspecting a cataract with the ophthalmoscope held at a distance from the eye, one must then approach closer and attempt to examine the fundus. Further useful information about the density of the cataract can be obtained in this way. It is generally true that if the observer can see in, then the patient can see out. If there is an obvious discrepancy between the clarity of the fundus and the visual acuity of the patient, then some other pathology may be suspected. Sometimes the patient may not have performed too well on subjective testing and such an error should be apparent when the fundus is viewed. Some types of cataract can be misleading in this respect and this applies particularly to those seen in highly myopic patients. Here there is sometimes a preponderance of nuclear sclerosis, which simply causes distortion of the fundus while the disc and macula may be seen quite clearly.

Findings on Slit-lamp Microscopy

A really detailed view of any cataract can be obtained with the slit-lamp. By adjusting the angle and size of the slit beam, various optical sections of the lens can be examined, revealing the exact morphology of the cataract. The presence of small vesicles under the anterior lens capsule may be seen as an early sign of senile cataract. Cataracts secondary to uveitis or to drugs may first appear as an opacity in the posterior subcapsular region. For optical reasons, an opacity in this region tends to interfere with reading vision at an early stage. Opacities in the lens may appear in a wide range of curious shapes and sizes, and earlier in this century there was a vogue for classifying them with Latin names which are now largely forgotten. Such a classification is of some help in deciding the cause of the cataract, although it may sometimes be misleading. Congenital cataracts are usually quite easily identified by their morphology, as also are some traumatic cataracts. When a unilateral cataract appears many years after a mild contusion injury, it may be difficult to distinguish this from an age-related one.

Other Important Signs

Certain other important signs need to be carefully elicited in a patient with cataracts. The pupil reaction is a particularly useful index of retinal function and it is not impaired by the densest of cataracts. A poor reaction may lead one to suspect age-related macular degeneration or chronic glaucoma, but a brisk pupil with a mature cataract might be described as a "surgeon's delight" because it indicates the likelihood of restoring good vision to a blind eye. The function of the peripheral retina can be usefully assessed by performing the light projection test. This entails seating the patient in a darkened room, covering one eye, and asking him or her to indicate, by pointing, the source of light from a torch positioned at different points in the peripheral field. Checking the pupil and the light projection test take a brief moment to perform and are by far the most important tests of retinal function when the retina cannot be seen directly. A number of other more sophisticated tests are available; ultrasonography, electroretinography and measurement of the visually evoked potential to mention some. Sometimes at least an area of the peripheral retina may be seen when the pupils have been dilated, and all cataract patients should be examined in this way before one embarks on more complex tests. A search for the signs of cataract thus involves a full routine eye examination including a measurement of the best spectacle correction.

Management

At the present time there is no effective medical treatment for cataract in spite of a number of claims over the years. A recent report has suggested that oral aspirin may delay the progress of cataract in female diabetics. Although this might be expected to have some effect on theoretical grounds any benefit is probably marginal. Occasionally patients claim that their cataracts seem to have cleared, but such fluctuation in density of the lens opacities has not been demonstrated in a scientific manner. Cataracts associated with galactosaemia are thought to clear under the influence of prompt treatment of the underlying problem.

Cataract is therefore essentially a surgical problem, and the management of a patient with cataract depends on deciding at what point the visual impairment of the patient justifies undergoing the risks of surgery. The cataract operation itself has been practised since pre-Christian times, and developments in recent years have made it safe and effective in a large proportion of cases. The operation entails removal of all the opaque lens fibres from within the lens capsule and replacing them with a clear plastic lens.

In the early part of this century the technical side of cataract surgery necessitated waiting for the cataract to become "ripe". Nowadays no such waiting is needed and it is theoretically possible to remove a clear lens. The decision to operate is based on whether the patient will see better afterwards. Modern cataract surgery can restore the vision in a remarkable way and patients often say that they have not seen so well for many years. Indeed many patients have quite reasonable vision without glasses but this cannot be guaranteed and, since the plastic lens implant gives a fixed focus, glasses will inevitably be needed for some distances. Probably the worst thing that can happen after the operation is infection leading to endophthalmitis and loss of the sight of the eye. Although this only occurs in about one out of a thousand cases the patient contemplating cataract surgery needs to be aware of the possibility. Before the operation, it is now a routine to measure the length of the eye and the corneal curvature. Knowing these two measurements, one can assess the strength of lens implant that is needed. When deciding on the strength of implant it is necessary to consider the other eye. The aim is usually to, make the two eyes optically similar because patients find it difficult to tolerate two different eyes.

When to Operate

Even though the decision to operate on a cataract must be made by the ophthalmic surgeon, the non-specialist general practitioner needs to understand the reasoning behind this decision. Elderly patients tend to forget what they have been told in the clinic and may not, for example, understand why cataract surgery is being delayed when macular degeneration is the main cause of visual loss. An operation is usually not required if the patient has not noticed any problem although sometimes the patient may deny the problem through some unexpressed fear. The requirements of the patient need to be considered; those of the chair-bound arthritic 80 year old who can still read small print quite easily are different from the younger business person who needs to be able to see a car number plate at 67 ft or 20.5 m in order to drive. The visual acuity by itself is not always a reliable guide. Some patients who have marked glare may need surgery with a visual acuity of 6/9 whereas others with less visual demands may be quite happy with a vision of 6/12 or 6/18. Early surgery may be needed to keep a joiner or bus driver at work for which good binocular vision is needed.

Age of the Patient

By itself, the age of the patient need have little influence on the decision to operate. Many people over the age of 100 years have had their cataracts successfully removed. The general health of the patient must be taken into account and this may influence one's decision in unexpected ways. Occasionally one is presented with a patient who has difficulty with balancing perhaps as a result of Ménière's disease or some other cause. The patient asks for cataract surgery in the hope that this will cure the problem. Unless the cataracts are advanced the result may be disappointing. Sometimes cataract surgery is requested in a nearly blind demented patient on the grounds that the dementia will improve with improvement of the vision. Although this occasionally happens, often the patient's mental state is made worse even though the sight is better. This raises some interesting ethical problems for the surgeon and relatives.

In the case of the child with congenital cataracts, the indications for surgery depend largely on the degree of opacification of the lens. An incomplete cataract may permit a visual acuity of 6/12 or 6/18 and yet the child may be able to read small print by exercising the large amount of available focusing power. Such a child could undergo normal schooling, and cataract surgery may never be required. A complete cataract in both eyes demands early surgery and this may be undertaken during the first few months of life. There is a high risk that one eye may become amblyopic in these young patients, even after cataract surgery.

Traumatic Cataract

This is usually a unilateral problem in a younger patient and sometimes the nature of the damage to the eye prevents the insertion of an intraocular lens. The patient may be left with no lens in the eye, a situation known as aphakia. Vision can be restored by a very strong convex spectacle lens but the difference between the two eyes makes it impossible to wear glasses. This is partly because everything looks much bigger with the corrected aphakic eye; the image on the retina is abnormally large. By wearing a contact lens on the cornea the optical problems may be solved but it is an unfortunate fact that patients with traumatic cataracts usually have working conditions which are unsuited to the wearing of a contact lens.

The Cataract Operation

Every medical student should witness at least one cataract operation during the period of training. It is an example of a classical procedure, which has been practised for 3000 years. The earliest method for dealing with cataract was known as couching. This entailed pushing the lens back into the vitreous where it was allowed to sink back into the fundus of the eye. Although this undoubtedly proved a simple and satisfactory procedure in some instances there is a tendency for the lens to set up a vigorous inflammatory reaction within the eye and subsequent loss of sight.

Modern cataract surgery was founded by the French surgeon Jacques Daviel in the eighteenth century. The operation that he devised involved seating the patient in a chair and making an incision around the lower half of the cornea. The lens was then removed through the opening. The results claimed were remarkable considering the technical difficulties that he must have encountered. Subsequently the procedure was facilitated by lying the patient down and making the incision around the upper part of the cornea where, in the postoperative period, it was protected by the upper eyelid. The use of local anaesthesia was introduced at the end of the nineteenth century and at the same time attempts were made to suture the cornea back into position. By the beginning of the twentieth century two methods had evolved for the actual removal of the lens. The safest way was to incise the anterior lens capsule and then wash out or express the opaque nucleus, preserving the posterior lens capsule as a protective wall against the bulging vitreous face. This is known as the extracapsular technique. The intracapsular cataract extraction became the standard operation of choice in most patients over the age of 50 years during the early part of the twentieth century. It involved removing the complete lens within its capsule and by this means avoided sub-

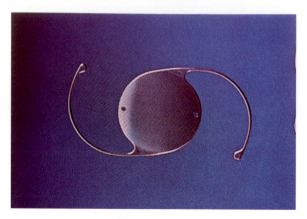

Fig. 11.3.   A typical plastic intraocular implant. There are different designs to suit different surgical techniques.

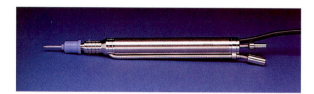

Fig. 11.4.   Type of probe used for phakoextraction of the opaque lens nucleus.

sequent operations to open up residual opaque posterior capsule.

Perhaps the most dramatic change in cataract surgery has occurred in the latter half of the twentieth century with the introduction of intraocular acrylic implants. Initially they were mostly employed with intracapsular surgery but a new technique for extracapsular surgery was then developed and found to be very successful with implants. Many different types and designs of intraocular lens have been used over the years. Figure 11.3 shows a commonly used type at the present day, but the trend is towards smaller incision surgery and the use of narrower implants and even foldable ones, which flip into position as they are being inserted into the eye. An important and widely used technique is phakoemulsification. Here the opaque lens nucleus is removed through a complex cannula, which breaks up the lens matter ultrasonically before sucking it from the eye (Figure 11.4).

Time Spent in Hospital

Many cataract operations are now done under local anaesthesia as day cases. General anaesthesia is pre-

ferred in younger patients and especially where there is a risk of straining or moving during the procedure as, for example, when the patient is deaf. An overnight stay is needed after a general anaesthetic in most cases. The elderly patient living alone with no relatives is also usually kept overnight in hospital but the trend is towards more and more day case work, dictated partly by economic reasons but also by safer surgery.

Convalescence

It is a fair generalisation to say that an eye requires two months for full healing to take place following a cataract operation. On the other hand, most of the healing takes place in the first two weeks. It is usual for patients to return to work after two weeks. After phakoemulsification glasses may be prescribed at this point but after larger incision surgery the prescription of new glasses is usually done after a month. The visual recovery is undoubtedly quicker after small incision surgery but the ultimate visual result is probably no better than when a larger incision is used. Presently the complication rate after small incision surgery and phakoemulsification may be slightly higher, but this may depend on the surgeon's experience. Most hospitals provide a "hand out" of do's and don'ts for the patients. The important thing is for the patient to avoid rubbing the eye and to seek immediate medical advice if the eye becomes painful. It is usual to instil antibiotic drops possibly combined with a steroid two or three times daily for two weeks.

Infection is the rare, but dreaded, complication and this is usually heralded by pain, redness, discharge and deterioration of vision. About 20% of patients develop opacification of the posterior lens capsule behind the implant after months or years. This is very simply cured by making an opening in the capsule with a special type of laser. This is a day case procedure, which requires no anaesthetic and takes two or three minutes. When corneal sutures have been used these may sometimes need to be removed and this can also be done on a "while you wait" basis in the outpatient department.

Summary

At primary care level it is important to be able to diagnose cataract but also to understand the benefits and risks of cataract surgery in order to be

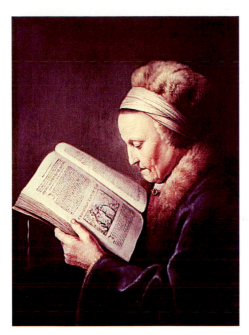

Fig. 11.5. An elderly person cannot read without glasses unless she is myopic. Myopia in the elderly may be due to cataract. ("Rembrandt's mother", with acknowledgement to Rijksmuseum-Stichting.)

able to give the patient advice as to when the cataract is bad enough to need an operation. An understanding of the meaning of aphakia and the optical consequences of an implant are also useful. Most patients who present with cataracts are diagnosed as having age-related cataracts and investigations as to the cause are limited to tests to exclude diabetes and to confirm that the patient is fit for surgery. An understanding of the symptoms of cataract is helped by understanding the meaning of index myopia.

Figure 11.5 is a final reminder of the signs and symptoms of cataract. An elderly woman would not normally be able to read small print without glasses and this lady's eyes must be abnormal. She may have inherited myopia allowing her to see near objects without the need for a presbyopic lens, but the myopia may also be index myopia, which in turn may be due to early cataract formation. Another cause of index myopia could be uncontrolled diabetes.

Glaucoma 12

The word "glaucoma" refers to the apparent grey–green colour of the eye suffering from an attack of acute narrow angle glaucoma. Nowadays the term has come to cover a group of eye diseases characterised by raised intraocular pressure. These diseases are quite distinct and the treatment in each case quite different. Glaucoma might be defined as a "pathological rise in the intraocular pressure sufficient enough to damage vision". This is to distinguish the normal elevation of intraocular pressure seen in otherwise normal individuals. Here we must consider what is meant by the "normal intraocular pressure".

Normal Intraocular Pressure

Measurement of the intraocular pressure in a large number of normal subjects reveals a normal distribution extending from pressures of 10–12 mmHg to pressures of 25–28 mmHg. The pattern of distribution fits a Gaussian curve, so that the majority of subjects have a pressure of about 16 mmHg. For clinical purposes it is necessary to set an arbitrary upper limit of normal. By and large, the eye can stand very low pressures remarkably well, but when the pressure is abnormally high, the circulation of blood through the eye becomes jeopardised and serious damage may ensue. For clinical purposes, an upper level of 21 mmHg is often accepted. Above this level, suspicions are raised and further investigations undertaken.

Maintenance of Intraocular Pressure

If the eye is to function as an effective optical instrument, it is clear that the intraocular pressure must be maintained at a constant level. At the same time, an active circulation of fluid through the globe is essential if the structures within it are to receive adequate nourishment. The cornea and sclera form a tough fibrous and unyielding envelope and within this an even pressure is maintained by a balance between the production and drainage of aqueous fluid.

Aqueous is produced by the ciliary epithelium by active secretion and ultrafiltration. A continuous flow is maintained through the pupil, when it reaches the angle of the anterior chamber.

On reaching the angle of the anterior chamber, aqueous passes through a grill known as the trabecular meshwork and then reaches a circular canal embedded in the sclera known as Schlemm's canal. This canal runs as a ring around the limbus (corneoscleral junction) and from it minute channels radiate outwards through the sclera to reach the episcleral circulation. These channels are known as aqueous veins and they transmit clear aqueous to the episcleral veins, which lie in the connective tissue underlying the conjunctiva. In actual fact, the proof of the route of drainage of aqueous can be verified by any medical student – it simply entails examining the white of the eye around the cornea with extreme care, using the high power of the slit-lamp microscope. After a time one can sometimes detect that some of the deeper veins convey parallel halves of blood and aqueous in the region beyond the junction of aqueous and episcleral vein.

The relative parts played by ciliary epithelium and trabecular meshwork in maintaining what is a remarkably constant intraocular pressure throughout life is not fully understood. It would appear that the production of aqueous is an active secretion whereas the drainage is more passive, although changing the tone of the ciliary muscle can alter the rate of drainage. In normal subjects the intraocular pressure does not differ in the two eyes by more than about 3 mmHg. Wider differences may lead one to suspect early glaucoma, especially if there is a family history of the disease. The normal intraocular pressure undergoes a diurnal variation, being highest in the early morning and gradually falling during the first half of the day. This diurnal change may become exaggerated as the first sign of glaucoma.

Measurement of Intraocular Pressure

The Schiotz tonometer (Figure 3.9) provides the simplest and cheapest way of measuring the intraocular pressure. It requires a certain expertise in its use but any training doctor with reasonable dexterity should become proficient with practice. The instrument consists of a central plunger, which moves freely within a hollow cylinder connected to a footpiece. The plunger is connected by a lever to a pointer on a dial.

To measure the pressure, the patient is asked to lie on a couch and a drop of local anaesthetic is instilled into the eyes. The eyelids of the left eye are held open gently, and without exerting any pressure on the eye, by the index finger and thumb of the left hand while the tonometer is lowered until the footpiece rides on the centre of the cornea. The plunger within the footpiece then impresses the cornea to a variable degree depending on the intraocular pressure. The amount of impression is indicted on the dial. The procedure is then repeated but this time the right finger and thumb keep open the right eyelids and the instrument is held in the left hand. The main disadvantage of this method of intraocular pressure measurement is that it gives inaccurate readings in eyes with abnormal scleral rigidity.

In ophthalmological clinics the Schiotz tonometer has been superseded by a more rapid and more accurate technique known as applanation tonometry. The applanation tonometer is supplied as an accessory to the slit-lamp microscope. The principle of applanation is as follows: when two balloons are pushed together so that the interface is a flat surface, then the pressure within the two balloons must be equal. By the same argument, when a fixed flat surface is pressed against a spherical surface such as the cornea, then at the point at which the spherical surface is exactly flattened the intraocular pressure

is equal to the pressure being applied. The applanation head is a small Perspex rod with a flattened end, which is fitted to a moveable arm. The tension applied to the moveable arm can be measured directly from a dial on the side of the instrument. The observer looks through the rod using the microscope of the slit-lamp, and the point at which exact flattening occurs can thus be gauged. For applanation tonometry, the patient is seated at the slit-lamp and not lying down but it is still necessary to instil a drop of local anaesthetic beforehand. Because the measurement of the intraocular pressure is such a basic requirement in any eye clinic, attempts have been made to introduce even more rapid and efficient devices. Perhaps the most ingenious to date is the tonometer which measures the indentation of the cornea in response to a puff of air by a photoelectric method. This air puff tonometer is less accurate than the Goldmann applanation tonometer. It is however good for screening.

Clinical Types of Glaucoma

It has been mentioned above that the word "glaucoma" refers to a group of diseases. For clinical purposes these may be subdivided into four:

1. Primary open angle glaucoma (P.O.A.G).
2. Acute closed angle glaucoma.
3. Secondary glaucoma.
4. Congenital glaucoma.

Primary Open Angle Glaucoma

The first important point to note about this disease is that it is very common, occurring in about 1% of the population over the age of 50 years. The second point is that the disease is inherited, and whereas the practice of screening the whole population for the disease is problematic in terms of finance, it is well worth screening the families of patients with the disease if those over the age of 40 are selected. This leads to the third point: That the incidence increases with age, being very rare under the age of 40. Primary open angle glaucoma is also termed chronic simple glaucoma, or simply chronic glaucoma. This insidious, potentially blinding disease affects those who are least likely to notice its onset, and elderly patients with advanced chronic open angle glaucoma are still seen from time to time in eye clinics.

Primary open angle glaucoma occurs more commonly in high myopes and diabetics; patients with Fuchs' corneal endothelial dystrophy and retinitis pigmentosa also have a higher incidence.

Pathogenesis and Natural History

Histologically there are remarkably few changes to account for the raised intraocular pressure, at least in the early stages of the disease. Subsequently, degenerative changes have been described in the juxta-canalicular trabecular meshwork, with endothelial thickening and oedema. In the lining of Schlemm's canal it has been shown that in the majority of cases the problem is one of inadequate drainage rather than excessive secretion of aqueous. In the untreated patient the chronically raised pressure leads to progressive damage to the eye and eventual blindness. The rate of progress of the disease varies greatly from individual to individual. It is possible for gross visual loss to occur within months, but usually the process takes five years. Younger eyes survive a raised pressure rather better than older eyes, which may already have circulatory problems. Very few eyes can withstand a pressure of 40 mmHg for more than a week or two or a pressure of 35 mmHg for more than a few months.

Chronic open angle glaucoma is nearly always bilateral, but often the disease begins in one eye, the other eye not becoming involved immediately. It is important to realise that the progress of chronic glaucoma can be arrested by treatment, but unfortunately many ophthalmologists experience the natural history of the disease by seeing neglected cases.

Symptoms

Most patients with chronic glaucoma have no symptoms. That is to say, the disease is insidious and is only detected at a routine eye examination either by an optometrist or ophthalmologist before the patient notices any visual loss. Occasionally younger patients notice a defect in their visual field but this is unusual. Unfortunately, the peripheral loss of visual field my pass unnoticed until it has reached an advanced stage.

Signs

The three cardinal signs are:

1. Raised intraocular pressure.
2. Cupping of the optic disc.
3. Visual field loss.

The intraocular pressure creeps up gradually to 30–35 mmHg, and it is this gradual rise which accounts for the lack of symptoms. Such a rise in intraocular pressure impairs the circulation of the optic disc, and the nerve fibres in this region become ischaemic. The combined effect of raised intraocular pressure and atrophy of nerve fibres results in gradual excavation of the physiological cup, and it is extremely useful to be able to identify this effect of raised intraocular pressure at an early stage. Figure 12.1 shows an optic disc undergoing various stages of pathological cupping. In the first instance the central physiological cup becomes enlarged, with its long axis arranged vertically. Notching of the neuroretinal rim of the optic disc tissue especially in the inferotemporal and superotemporal region is common. The edge of the optic disc cup corresponds to the bend in the blood vessels as they cross the disc surface. In some eyes the area of pallor may correspond to the cup whilst in others the cup is larger

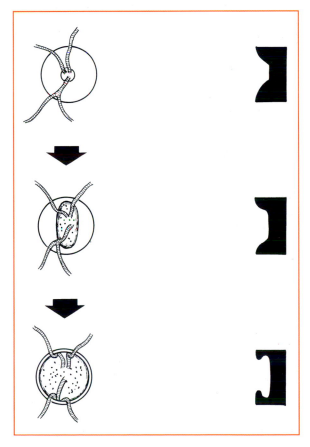

Fig. 12.1. The effect of glaucoma on the optic disc.

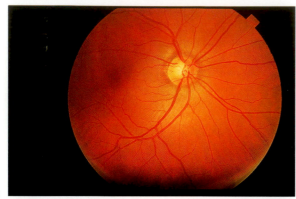

a

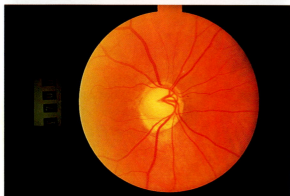

b

Fig. 12.2. **a** Glaucomatous cupping of the disc early cupping; **b** advanced cupping.

than the area of pallor. It is particularly useful to observe the way in which the vessels enter and leave the nerve head (Figure 12.2). A flame-shaped haemorrhage at the disc margin may be seen. Localised loss of retinal nerve fibres may be observed especially with a red-free light.

The changes in the visual field can be deduced from observing the disc and from considering the arrangement of the nerve fibres in the eye. If we gaze fixedly with one eye at a spot on the wall and then move a small piece of paper on the end of a paper clip, or even the end of our index finger, in such a manner as to explore our peripheral field, it is soon possible to locate the blind spot. In the case of the right eye, this is found slightly to the right of the point of fixation because it represents the projected position of the optic nerve head in the right eye. The blind spot is rounded and about 8–12° lateral to and slightly below the level of fixation. It has already been mentioned that the glaucomatous disc is initially excavated above and below so that the patient with early glaucoma has a blank area in the visual field extending in an arcuate manner from the blind spot above and below fixation. This typical pattern of field loss is known as the arcuate scotoma. If the glaucoma remains uncontrolled, this scotoma extends peripherally and centrally. It can be seen that even at this stage the central part of the field may be well preserved and the patient may still be able to read the smallest letters on the Snellen test chart. If the field loss is allowed to progress further, the patient becomes blind.

Treatment

For many years the mainstay in the treatment of primary open angle glaucoma has been the use of miotic drops. The miotic of choice was pilocarpine, starting with the 1% solution and increasing to 4% if needed. Recently the treatment has undergone a minor revolution as the result of the introduction of the β-blockers e.g. timolol, levubunolol (Betagan) and betaxolol (Betoptic) as well as many other types of topical medication (see Table 12.1). Pilocarpine itself is very effective in reducing the intraocular pressure. After about half an hour from the moment of instillation, the pupil becomes small and the patient experiences dimming of the vision, aching over the eyebrow and a spasm of accommodation which blurs the distance vision. At the same time the intraocular pressure in the majority of fresh cases of chronic glaucoma falls to within the normal range. After about 4 h the intraocular pressure begins to rise again and the side-effects wear off. This, of

Table 12.1.   Topical glaucoma medication

Drug type	Examples	Mechanism of action
β-Blockers	Timolol Betaxolol Levubunolol Carteolol	Reduce aqueous production
Cholinergics	Parasympathominetics Pilocarpine Anticholinesterases Phospholine Iodide	Increase aqueous outflow via trabecular meshwork
Adrenergic agonists α_2-Agonist	Adrenaline and Prodrug (Dipivefrine) Brimonidine	Decrease aqueous production and increase uveoscleral outflow
Carbonic anhydrase inhibitors	Dorzolomide	Reduce aqueous production
Prostaglandins	Latanoprost (prostaglandin-2-alpha)	Increased uveoscleral outflow

course, means that a further drop of pilocarpine must be instilled if good control is to be continued. It is here that we find the most difficult problem of treatment. Human nature is such that drops are rarely instilled four times daily on a regular basis, although patients are genuinely anxious to preserve their eyesight. It is fortunate that timolol and other β-blockers are effective over a 12-h period and need to be instilled only twice daily. As an ocular hypotensive agent these are probably not quite as effective as pilocarpine, but many cases of chronic glaucoma are now satisfactorily controlled by them and furthermore the drug may be used in combination with pilocarpine. β-Blockers have the further advantage that they do not cause any miosis. The main side-effects of β-blockers are bronchospasm, reduced cardiac contractability and bradycardia. They are therefore contraindicated in patients with chronic obstructive airway disease, heart block, hypotension and bradycardia. Anticholinesterase drugs such as echothiopate (phospholine iodine) and demecarium bromide (Humorsol) are also very effective ocular hypotensive agents when administered in drop form. However, their use tends to be reserved for aphakic glaucoma because they are inclined to increase the rate of formation of cataracts, and iris cysts; rarely they may also predispose to retinal detachment. Systemic effects have been noted in some patients undergoing general anaesthesia combined with the use of succinylcholine: "scoline apnoea".

The cholinergic drugs such as pilocarpine and the anticholinesterase drugs (such as echothiopate iodide) act by increasing the rate of outflow of aqueous, whereas timolol is thought to inhibit the production of aqueous. Adrenaline drops also have the effect of reducing aqueous production and they have been in use for some years as a supplement to pilocarpine. However, their effect is not very powerful and they tend to cause chronic dilatation of the conjunctival vessels in some patients as well as the deposition of pigment in the conjunctiva and subconjunctival fibrosis.

Oral acetazolamide is only occasionally used in chronic glaucoma because of its long-term side-effects. Acetazolamide (Diamox) is a carbonic anhydrase inhibitor, which was introduced many years ago as a diuretic. Its diuretic action is not very well sustained, but it is a potent drug for reducing intraocular pressure. If a normal subject takes a 250–500 mg tablet of the drug, the eye becomes very soft after about an hour. Every patient taking acetazolamide experiences paraesthesiae of the hands

and feet and some complain of gastric symptoms. Occasionally patients become lethargic or even confused. Young patients, particularly young males, may suffer renal colic. It should be pointed out that these more serious side-effects are rare, and long-term acetazolomide is still sometimes used when no other means of controlling the intraocular pressure is available.

Newer glaucoma medications include Latanoprost, Dorzolamide and Brimonidine. Latanoprost is a prostaglandin, which produces its intraocular pressure lowering effect through increased uveoscleral outflow. It appears to be superior to β-blockers in its hypotensive effect. The main side-effects are slight conjunctival congestion and increased iris pigmentation in some patients with mixed coloured irises.

Dorzolamide (Trusopt) is the first topically administered carbonic anhydrase inhibitor. Its pressure lowering effect is inferior to that of timolol.

Brimonidine (Alphagan) is an α_2-adrenergic agonist, which decreases aqueous production and also increases the uveoscleral outflow. It has a pressure lowering effect comparable to that of timolol. It has the advantage of not having any effect on the respiratory system. It can therefore be used in patients with obstructive airway disease.

If the intraocular pressure remains uncontrolled by safe medical treatment and there is evidence of continued loss of visual field, then surgical treatment is indicated. A large number of operations have been devised for the management of chronic open angle glaucoma and most of these entail allowing the aqueous to drain subconjunctivally through an artificial opening made in the sclera. The operation, which is usually preferred at the present time,

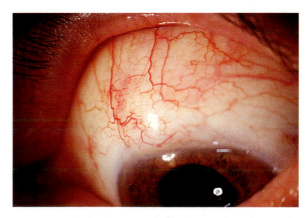

Fig. 12.3. Trabeculectomy bleb.

is the "trabeculectomy". In this operation a superficial "trapdoor" of sclera is raised and the deeper layer, including the trabecular meshwork, is removed. The trapdoor is then sewn back into position. Aqueous drains around the edge of this scleral flap into the subconjunctiva (Figure 12.3). Although most of these operations may reduce the intra-ocular pressure very effectively and often for many years, they all tend to increase the rate of formation of cataract. This and the risk of postoperative endophthalmitis are the main reasons why surgery is usually not considered the first line of treatment in chronic open angle glaucoma by most ophthalmologists.

Normal Tension Glaucoma (NTG)

This condition is similar to POAG except that the intraocular pressure is within normal limits, for instance 21 mmHg or less at the initial and subsequent visits. The condition is probably due to low perfusion pressure at the optic nerve head so that the nerve head is susceptible to damage at normal intraocular pressure.

Certain conditions that may mimic NTG include compressive lesions of the optic nerve and chiasma, carotid ischaemia and congenital optic disc anomalies.

Treatment of NTG aims to reduce intraocular pressure to 12 mmHg or less.

Management

Most eye units now run special clinics for dealing with glaucoma patients. From what has been said, it should be clear that patients with chronic glaucoma require much time and attention. Initially the nature of the disease must be explained and patients must realise that the treatment is to arrest the progress of the condition and not to cure it. Furthermore, any visual loss that occurs is irretrievable, so that regular follow-up visits are essential for checking the intra-ocular pressure and carefully assessing the visual fields.

The initial treatment is a single topical agent – usually a β-blocker (unless contraindicated). The second line treatments of choice are Brimonidine, Latanoprost or Trusopt.

Acute Closed Angle Glaucoma

This condition is less common than chronic open angle glaucoma, comprising about 5% of all cases of primary glaucoma. It is a much more dramatic condition than the chronic disease and fits in more closely with the popular lay idea of "glaucoma". It tends to affect a slightly younger age group than chronic glaucoma and only occurs in predisposed individuals. There is a particular type of eye, which is liable to develop acute glaucoma: this is a small hypermetropic eye with a shallow anterior chamber. One never meets a myope with acute glaucoma. This fact bears a special importance when attempting to diagnose a subacute attack.

Pathogenesis and Natural History

The eye, which is going to develop closed angle glaucoma, has a shallow anterior chamber and is hypermetropic. There is forward bowing of the iris which is more evident in these individuals and the corneal diameter is smaller than in normal eyes. Another factor is the gradual but slight increase in size of the lens, which takes place with ageing. The rise in intraocular pressure, which occurs, is due to occlusion of the angle by the iris root and it may be precipitated by dilating the pupil. An uncontrolled acute attack of glaucoma can lead to rapid and permanent loss of the sight of the affected eye. Although it is known that occasionally patients recover spontaneously from such an attack, they may be left with chronic angle closure and a picture similar to that of chronic open angle glaucoma. About half the patients with closed angle glaucoma will develop a similar problem in the other eye if steps are not taken to prevent this, and it will be seen that prophylactic treatment for the other eye is now the rule.

Symptoms

The subacute attack. Here it might be helpful to consider a typical patient, who might be a male or female, aged about 50 years. Such a patient would have a moderate degree of hypermetropia and rather a narrow gap between iris and cornea as shown by the shallow anterior chamber. During the autumn months, this patient's pupil might be noted to be slightly wider, as one might expect with the dimmer illumination and one evening the pupil dilates sufficiently to allow the iris root to nudge across the angle and obstruct the flow of aqueous. Immediately the intraocular pressure rises acutely, perhaps to 30 or 40 mmHg and pain is felt over the eye. At the same time the acute rise of pressure causes the cornea to become oedematous. Since it is evening, the patient observes that streetlights when viewed through the oedematous cornea appear to have coloured rings around them, as if they were being viewed through frosted glass. At this point the patient retires to bed and on sleeping the pupil becomes small and the intraocular pressure rise is relieved. After several of these attacks, the patient may seek attention from the family doctor. Patients present as healthy people with evening headaches associated with blurring of the vision and they are wearing moderately thick convex lenses in their spectacles. Subacute glaucoma is easily missed, partly because it is rare amongst the large number of sufferers from headache. If attention is not sought at this stage or if the diagnosis is missed, then one evening the acute attack develops.

The acute attack. After a number of subacute attacks an irreversible turn of events may occur. The iris root becomes congested, raising the intraocular pressure further and producing further congestion. The headache becomes much worse and the vision becomes seriously impaired. The doctor, who may be called in the following morning, is confronted with a patient who is nauseated and vomiting and at first sight an acute abdominal problem may be suspected until the painful red eye should make the diagnosis obvious. Sometimes acute glaucoma does not cause much pain or nausea and in these cases the physical signs in the eye become especially important (Figure 12.4).

Signs

The most obvious physical sign is the semidilated fixed pupil. The iris and the constricting sphincter muscle of the pupil are damaged by the raised intraocular pressure. The pupil is not able to constrict and after a day or two the iris becomes depigmented, taking on the grey atrophic colour, which gave glaucoma its name. Prompt and effective treatment should prevent any damage to the iris. The eye is red and a pink grill of engorged deeper capillaries is seen around the corneal margin; this important sign, as opposed to conjunctival inflammation is known as ciliary injection. Corneal oedema can usually be detected without optical aids by observing the lack of lustre in the eye and any attempts to assess the hardness of the eye by palpating it through the eyelids will elicit another sign, that of tenderness of the globe. The visual acuity may be reduced to "hand movements" in a severe attack. There are two rather subtle signs that often persist permanently after the acute attack has been resolved. The first is the presence of a white, irregular microscopic deposit just deep to the anterior surface of the lens, and the second is the presence of whorl atrophy in the iris. The pattern of the iris becomes twisted as if the sphincter has been rotated slightly. Both these signs may provide useful evidence of a previous attack, which has resolved spontaneously.

Measurement of the intraocular pressure at this point may reveal a reading of 70 mmHg or more. Very gentle palpation of the globe is usually enough to confirm that the eye has the consistency of a brick, especially when the pressures of the two eyes are compared. It should be realised that digital palpation of the globe can be very misleading and the method cannot be used to detect smaller rises in intraocular pressure with any degree of reliability (Table 12.2).

Examination of the other eye will reveal a shallow anterior chamber. Shining a focused beam of light obliquely through the cornea and noting the width of the gap between where the light strikes the cornea and where it strikes the iris can assess the depth of the anterior chamber. After inspecting a few normal eyes in this way, the observer can soon learn when an anterior chamber is abnormally shallow. This facility is important to anyone who intends to instil

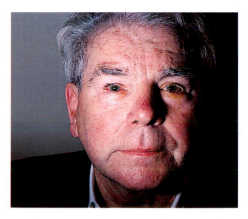

Fig. 12.4.   Acute angle closure glaucoma.

Table 12.2.   Signs of acute glaucoma

- Ciliary injection
- Semi-dilated oval pupil
- Corneal oedema
- Tenderness of globe
- Poor vision
- Shallow anterior chambers
- Hard eye

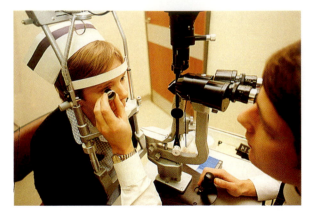

Fig. 12.5.   Preparing for gonioscopy.

mydriatic drops into an eye A shallow anterior chamber does not contraindicate mydriatic drops but it does indicate the need for extreme caution and care that the pupil is afterwards restored to its normal size. The angle of the anterior chamber itself is not exposed to direct inspection and it can only be seen through a gonioscope (Figure 12.5). This instrument is a contact lens with a mirror mounted on it and through it the width of the angle can be estimated. If the angle is open, the various structures adjacent to the iris root and inner surface of the peripheral cornea can be identified. Gonioscopy forms a routine part of the examination of any patient with glaucoma although in acute narrow angle glaucoma the presence of a closed angle can often be presumed by the presence of the other physical signs. Where there is any doubt, it may be necessary to apply a drop of hypertonic glycerol to the cornea to clear the oedema before applying the gonioscope.

The sooner closed angle glaucoma is diagnosed and treated then, the better are the results of treatment. Unfortunately, it is in the early subacute stage of the disease that the diagnosis may be difficult. A number of provocative tests have been devised for the patient who presents with suspicious symptoms but a normal intraocular pressure. The simplest test is the "dark room test": The patient's intraocular pressure is measured before he or she is seated in a darkened room for half an hour. The intraocular pressure is again measured immediately after this, and a rise in pressure of more than 5 mmHg may be taken to be significant. Certain drugs can have a similar effect by having a mildly mydriatic action when taken by mouth. The phenothiazines have been incriminated in this respect. Of course, such

drugs will have no adverse effect on patients who have already been treated and identified as cases of narrow or closed angle glaucoma. Only in unsuspected cases of subacute narrow angle glaucoma is there a real risk of precipitating an acute attack.

Treatment

Acute narrow angle glaucoma is a surgical problem and any patient suffering from the condition requires urgent admission to hospital. To do less than this is to undertreat the condition and run the risk of producing chronic narrow angle glaucoma. On admission the affected eye is treated with intensive miotic drops. A typical regime would be the application of pilocarpine 4% every minute for 5 min then every 5 min for an hour followed by instillation every hour. This treatment is supported by an injection of acetazolomide. If the renal function is unimpaired, acetazolomide may be given intravenously (usually 500 mg) followed by an oral dose of 250 mg four times a day. Topical β-blockers and/or trusopt and reduction of inflammation and iris congestion by topical steroids may help achieve a quicker lowering of intraocular pressure. In many cases these measures relieve the acute attack within hours. However, some patients may require an intravenous infusion of mannitol. During this period the patient is kept in bed and analgesics are given if required. It is important that the other eye is also treated with pilocarpine 2% four times a day in order to prevent a second disaster.

Once the intraocular pressure has been controlled, the cure is maintained by performing a peripheral iridectomy. By this simple operation, a small triangular hole is made in the peripheral iris. This allows the bulging iris bombe to sink backwards like a punctured ship's sail and is a sure means of preventing further acute attacks. The following week it is usual to carry out a similar prophylactic operation on the fellow eye although some surgeons may prefer to operate on both eyes at the same time. In some patients the angle of the anterior chamber remains partially occluded by peripheral adhesions from the iris. In these cases a simple peripheral iridectomy may not be adequate and it may be necessary to carry out a drainage operation such as a trabeculectomy. Most patients with acute narrow angle glaucoma are cured by surgery, although a small proportion develops cataracts in later years. The prognosis in adequately treated narrow angle glaucoma is therefore very good, but in the absence of treatment the result is disastrous.

The treatment of narrow angle glaucoma has undergone a small revolution over the past few years. This is because a new generation of lasers has appeared which make it possible to perforate the iris quite simply. The YAG (yttrium–aluminium–garnet) laser seems to have successfully replaced surgical iridectomy in most cases. A special contact lens is used to focus the laser on the peripheral iris. Usually more than one iridectomy is made in each. Postoperatively steroids and pupil dilatation are required.

Secondary Glaucoma

The intraocular pressure may become raised as the result of a number of different disease processes in the eye quite apart from the causes of primary glaucoma, which have just been described.

Secondary to Vascular Disease in the Eye

Central retinal vein thrombosis. This is a common cause of sudden blurring of the vision of one eye in the elderly. The retinal veins can be seen to be dilated and surrounded by haemorrhages. In some cases, recovery is marred by a rise in intraocular pressure, which is delayed for about three months. The prompt appearance of this very painful complication has given it the name of "hundred-day glaucoma". This type of glaucoma is usually difficult to control and even surgical measures may prove ineffective. A typical feature is the appearance of a vascular membrane over the anterior surface of the iris and sometimes the angle of the anterior chamber. This vascularised tissue lends a pinkish hue to the iris and is termed rubeosis iridis. Patients with a central retinal vein thrombosis followed by secondary glaucoma have another problem because there is a recognised association between chronic open angle glaucoma and central retinal vein occlusion. This means that some patients who present with an occluded vein are found to have chronic glaucoma in the other eye.

Diabetes. Patients with severe diabetic retinopathy may also develop rubeosis iridis and secondary glaucoma. The vascular occlusive features of diabetic eye disease give it many resemblances to central retinal vein thrombosis and the secondary glaucoma which develops is also very resistant to medical treatment. Panretinal laser photocoagulation when applied early causes regression of the rubeosis. The ultimate outcome is sometimes a blind and painful eye, which has to be removed.

Secondary to Uveitis

During an attack of acute iridocyclitis the intraocular pressure is often below normal because the production of aqueous by the ciliary body is reduced. When the normal production of aqueous is resumed it may induce a rise in pressure because the outflow channels have been obstructed by inflammatory exudate. This type of secondary glaucoma responds to vigorous treatment of the iridocyclitis, and here it is essential to dilate and not constrict the pupil and to apply steroid treatment. Acetazolamide and topical β-blockers, for example Timolol and Betagan, may also be required. The type of secondary glaucoma, which develops after the iridocyclitis of herpes zoster infections, can be particularly insidious. The intraocular pressure may remain high without obvious pain and with relatively slight inflammatory changes in the eye. Secondary glaucoma usually responds well to treatment and once the underlying inflammation has subsided the eye returns to normal.

In iridocyclitis glaucoma may also be due to pupil block (inability of aqueous to pass from the posterior to anterior chamber) because of posterior synechiae (adhesions between the iris and lens). Treatment is YAG laser iridotomy.

Secondary to Tumours

Malignant melanoma of the choroid and retinoblastoma may cause glaucoma. The raised intraocular pressure can be an important diagnostic feature when a suspected lesion is seen in the fundus. When a patient presents with a blind glaucomatous eye the possibility of malignancy must always be in the back of one's mind.

Secondary to Trauma

Trauma may precipitate a rise in intraocular pressure in a number of different ways. Sometimes, especially in children, bleeding may occur into the anterior chamber after a contusion injury. This can seriously obstruct the flow of aqueous both through the pupil and into the angle. Such an episode of bleeding may occur on the second or third day after the injury, turning a slight event into a very serious problem. On other occasions a contusion injury may cause splitting or recession of the angle which is associated with glaucoma. The iridocyclitis, which follows perforating injuries, tends to be complicated by glaucoma and the ophthalmologist must be constantly aware of such a complication.

Drug-induced Glaucoma

Local and also systemic steroids can cause a rise in intraocular pressure and this is more likely to occur in patients with a family history of glaucoma. Steroid glaucoma is now a well-recognised phenomenon and "steroid reactors" can be identified by measuring the intraocular pressure before and after instilling a drop of dexamethasone. The less potent steroids, hydrocortisone and prednisolone, are less likely to cause this problem and new steroids such as Clobethasone are now being produced with the claim that they have the anti-inflammatory effect of dexamethasone but no effect on intraocular pressure.

The possibility of inducing primary closed angle glaucoma by drugs has already been mentioned.

Secondary to Abnormalities in the Lens

A cataractous lens may become hypermature and swell up, pushing the iris diaphragm forwards and obstructing the angle of the anterior chamber. This is referred to as phacomorphic glaucoma. Removing the lens relieves the situation. Phacolytic glaucoma occurs when a mature cataract causes a type of uveitis. This is thought to result from leakage of lens proteins through the lens capsule. A dislocated or subluxated lens, either the result of trauma or as a congenital abnormality, can be associated with a rise in intraocular pressure.

Local and systemic steroids can cause a rise in intraocular pressure and this is more likely to occur in patients with a family history of glaucoma. Steroid glaucoma is now a well-recognised phenomenon and "steroid reactors" can be identified by measuring the intraocular pressure before and after instilling a drop of steroid. The less potent steroids, hydrocortisone and prednisolone, are less likely to cause this problem and new steroids are now being produced with the claim that they have minimal effect on the intraocular pressure. The possibility of inducing an attack of acute glaucoma by drugs has already been mentioned.

Congenital or Developmental Glaucoma

These glaucomas occur in eyes in which an anomaly present at birth produces an intraocular pressure rise.

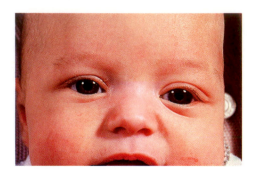

Fig. 12.6.   Congenital glaucoma: note the enlarged left cornea (with acknowledgement to Mr R. Gregson).

This type of glaucoma is extremely rare and it is often, though not always, inherited. This means that the affected child may be brought to the ophthalmologist by the parents because they are aware of the condition in the family. Children may be born with raised intraocular pressure and for these cases the prognosis is not so good as in those where the pressure rise does not occur until after the first few months of life.

In primary developmental glaucoma the glaucoma is due to defective development of the angle of the anterior chamber, and gonioscopy shows that the normal features of the angle are obscured by a pinkish membrane. Raised intraocular pressure in infancy has a dramatic effect because it causes enlargement of the globe. This can best be observed by noting an increase in the corneal diameter. The enlarged eye has given the condition the name of buphthalmos or "bull's eye" (Figure 12.6). Other important signs are photophobia and corneal oedema. The diagnosis is confirmed by an examination under anaesthesia, which includes measuring the corneal diameters and the intraocular pressure. Surgical treatment is nearly always required and this involves passing a fine knife through the peripheral cornea so that the point reaches the opposite angle of the anterior chamber. Once in the angle, it is moved gently to and fro to open up the embryonic tissue which covers the trabecular meshwork (goniotomy). The other (or secondary) developmental glaucomas include the rubella syndrome, aniridia, mesodermal dysgenesis, Peter's anomaly and the phacomatoses where the intraocular pressure rise is associated with other ocular and systemic developmental anomalies.

Retinal Detachment

Detachment of the retina signifies an inward separation of the sensory part of the retina from the retinal pigment epithelium (RPE). There is an accumulation of fluid in the space between the neural retina and the RPE known as subretinal fluid (Figure 13.1). The retina bulges inwards like the collapsed bladder of a football. Once detached, the retina can no longer function and in humans it tends to remain detached, unless treatment is available.

Although the condition is relatively rare in the general population, it is important for several reasons. First, it is a blinding condition which can be treated very effectively and often dramatically by surgery. Second, retinal detachment may on occasions be the first sign of malignant disease in the eye. Finally, nowadays the condition may often be prevented by prophylaxis in predisposed eyes.

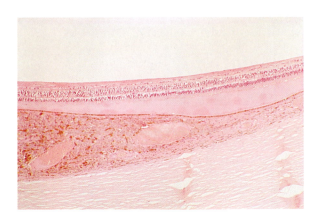

Fig. 13.1. Histology of retinal detachment showing the location of subretinal fluid. This eye has an underlying choroidal melanoma.

Incidence

Retinal detachment is rare in the general population but an eye unit serving a population of 500,000 might expect to be looking after three or four cases a week. It can be seen, therefore, that a doctor in general practice might see a case once in every two or three years, especially if we consider that some retinal detachment patients go directly to eye casualty departments without seeking non-specialist advice. Although children are sometimes affected, the incidence increases with age and reaches a maximum in the 50–60-year age group. There is a smaller peak in the mid-20s to 30s due to traumatic detachments in young males.

Certain groups of people are especially liable to develop detachment of the retina: severely shortsighted patients have been shown to have an incidence as high as 3.5% and about 1% of aphakic patients have detachments.

In just under one-quarter of cases, if there is no intervention, the other eye becomes affected at a later date. This means that the sound eye must be examined with great care in every instance.

Pathogenesis

There is an embryological explanation for retinal detachment in that the separating layers open up a potential space which existed during the early development of the eye as described previously (Chapter 2). The inner lining of the eye develops as two layers. In its earliest stages of development, the eye is seen as an outgrowth of the forebrain, the optic vesicle, the cavity of which is continuous with that of the forebrain. The vesicle becomes invaginated to form the optic cup, and the two-layered cup becomes the two layered lining of the adult eye. Anteriorly in the eye the two layers line the inner surface of the iris and ciliary body. Posterior to the ciliary body the outer of the two layers remains as a single layer of pigmented cells, known as the pigment epithelium. The inner of the two layers becomes many cells thick and develops into the sensory retina. In the adult the sensory retina is closely linked, both physically and metabolically, with the pigment epithelium and, in particular the production of visual pigment relies on this juxtaposition. When the retina becomes detached and the sensory retina is separated from the pigment epithelium, the retina can no longer function and the sight is lost in the detached area. Both pigment epithelium and sensory retina are included in the term "retina" and in this sense "retinal detachment" is a misnomer.

The retina receives its nourishment from two sources: the inner half deriving its blood supply from the central retinal artery, and the outer half from the choroid. The important foveal region is supplied mainly by the choroid. When the retina is detached, the central retinal artery remains intact and continues to supply it since it is also detached with it. The outer half of the retina is deprived of nourishment, being separated from pigment epithelium and choroid. Eventually degenerative changes appear, the fovea being affected at an early stage. It is interesting that after surgical replacement the retina regains much of its function during the first few days but further recovery may occur over as long a period as one or even two years.

Classification

Detachment of the retina may occur as the result of:

● Holes in the sensory retina due to either to degeneration (spontaneous) or to trauma (rhegmatogenous retinal detachment).

● Traction from within: fibrous strands may form in the vitreous and subsequently contract causing the sensory retina to be tented up from the RPE. This is seen after penetrating eye injury or in proliferative diabetic retinopathy (tractional retinal detachment).

● Pressure from outside: an expanding choroidal tumour is usually associated with retinal detachment; very rarely, inflammatory exudate may be the cause. The fluid gains access to the subretinal space through damaged RPE (exudative retinal detachment).

Rhegmatogenous Retinal Detachment

The Formation of Holes in the Retina

It was noticed as long ago as 1853, only a short time after the invention of the ophthalmoscope, that many detached retinae have minute holes in them, but it was not until the 1920s that the full significance of these holes as the basic cause of the detachment became realised. The holes may be single or multiple and are more commonly situated in the anterior or more peripheral part of the retina. They are usually horseshoe shaped, though sometimes rounded. In order to understand how these tears or holes occur, it is necessary to understand something of retinal degeneration and vitreous changes.

Retinal degeneration

When examining the peripheral retina of otherwise normal subjects, it is surprising to find that from time to time there are quite striking degenerative changes. Perhaps this is not so surprising when one considers that the retinal arteries are end arteries and these changes occur in the peripheral parts of the retina supplied by the distal part of the circulation. Different types of degeneration have been described and named and certain types are recognised as being the precursors to hole formation. The most important degenerations are lattice, white without pressure and retinoschisis. Peripheral retinal degenerations are more commonly seen in myopic eyes, especially in association with Marfan's and Ehlers–Danlos syndromes and Stickler's disease (see Further reading at the end of the book).

The Vitreous

The normal vitreous is a clear gel, which occupies most of the inside of the eye. Its consistency is similar to that of raw white of egg and, being a gel, it takes up water and salts. It is made up of a meshwork of collagen fibres whose interspaces are filled with molecules of hyaluronic acid. The vitreous is adherent to the retina at the ora serrata (junction of ciliary body and retina) and around the optic disc and macula. If we move our eyes, the vitreous moves, and, being restrained by its attachment, swings back to its original position again. The vitreous is usually perfectly transparent but most people become aware of small particles of cellular debris, which can be observed against a clear background such as a blue sky or an X-ray screen. These particles can be seen to move slowly with eye movement and appear to have momentum, just as one would expect if one considers the way the vitreous moves.

These vitreous floaters are commonplace and tend to increase in number as the years pass. They often become more evident to the individual when under stress; the anxious student may observe a floater following the gaze across the page of a book and this may set in train a series of worries about possible eye disease. Patients quite commonly present with this symptom when their real problem is anxiety or stress. But the vitreous undergoes a more dramatic change with age. Often in the late 50s, it becomes more fluid and collapses from above, coming away from its normal position against the retina and eventually lying as a contracted mobile gel in the inferior and anterior part of the cavity of the globe. The rest of the globe is occupied by clear fluid. When this happens the patient may complain of something floating in front of the vision and also the appearance of flashing lights. This is because the mobile shrunken vitreous sometimes causes slight traction on the retina. As a rule, the same symptoms are then experienced subsequently in the other eye. It is very common to find a detached vitreous in an elderly person's eye in the absence of any symptoms. This then is the condition known as posterior vitreous detachment (PVD). It is common and usually of no pathological significance. One must be careful about the use of the term "detachment" in front of the patient because for many people this means only one thing, a detached retina.

Unfortunately it is true that when the vitreous detaches it may, on rare occasions, cause the formation of a retina tear or hole, possibly at a point of pre-existing abnormal attachment of vitreous to retina. The retinal tear associated with PVD is normally in the superior fundus. There may be a vitreous haemorrhage. Occasionally PVD may cause avulsion of a peripheral retinal blood vessel without a retinal tear.

Signs and Symptoms of Retinal Hole Formation

Let us now consider a typical patient, possibly a myope in the middle 50s either male or female, who suddenly experiences the symptoms of "flashes and floaters", sometimes spontaneously or sometimes after making a sudden head movement. The symptoms are similar to those produced by a vitreous detachment but tends to be more pronounced and obvious to the patient. Proper interpretation of such symptoms can save sight and they will therefore be considered in more detail.

Flashes ("Photopsiae")

When questioned, the patient usually says that these are probably present all the time but are only noticeable in the dark. They seem to be especially apparent before going to sleep at night. The flashes are usually seen in the peripheral part of the visual field. They must be distinguished from the flashes seen in migraine, which are quite different and are usually followed by headache. The migrainous subject tends to see zig-zag lines, which spread out from the centre of the field and last for about 10 min. Elderly patients with a defective vertebrobasilar circulation may describe another type of photopsia in which the flashing lights tend to occur only with neck movements or after bending.

Floaters

It has already been explained that black spots floating in front of the vision are commonplace but often called to our attention by anxious patients. When the spots are large and appear suddenly, they may be of pathological significance. For some reason patients often refer to them as tadpoles or frog-spawn or even a spider's web. It is the combination of these symptoms with flashing lights that makes it important.

Flashes and floaters appear because the vitreous has tugged on the retina producing the sensation of light and often when the tear appears there is a slight bleeding into the vitreous, causing the black spots. When clear-cut symptoms of this kind appear, they must not be overlooked. The eyes must be examined fully until the tear in the retina is found. Sometimes a small tear in the retina is accompanied by a large vitreous haemorrhage and thus sudden loss of vision. In such a case the proper treatment is rest for two or three days to reduce the risk of further haemorrhage, after which the retinal tear can often be seen and then treated. Other causes of vitreous haemorrhage such as proliferative retinopathy as in retinal vein occlusions, sickle-cell retinopathy, and diabetes, retinal vasculitis, retinal macroaneurysm or trauma, must be considered.

Traumatic Holes

A perforating injury of the eye can produce a tear at any point in the retina, but contusion injuries commonly produce tears in the extreme retinal periphery and in the lower temporal quadrant or the superior nasal quadrant. This is because the lower temporal quadrant of the globe is most exposed to injury from a flying missile such as squash ball. The threatened eye makes an upward movement as the lids attempt to close. Tears of this kind often take the form of a dialysis, the retina being torn away in an arc from the ora serrata. Warning symptoms in these patients are usually masked by the symptoms of the original injury and they tend to present some months, or occasionally years, after the original injury with the symptoms of a retinal detachment. This is unfortunate because the tear can be treated if it is located before the detachment occurs.

When the presence of a retinal tear is suspected, the pupils of both eyes must be widely dilated and the fundi examined by direct and indirect ophthalmoscopy. The triple mirror gonioscope is also used to obtain a microscopic view of the peripheral fundus. At this stage a drawing is usually made of the location of any tears or weak areas. Many tears can be found with the direct ophthalmoscope alone, but using this instrument for the peripheral fundus demands some extra practice.

Studies on post-mortem eyes show that some patients have flat retinal tears and do not develop retinal detachments. Probably only a small percentage of tears lead to a detachment, but certain types of tear are very likely to cause trouble. These are: tears with symptoms, tears that are large, and tears that are situated in the upper part of the retina. However, all retinal tears must be suspect and referred for specialist assessment.

Signs and Symptoms of Retinal Detachment

Once a retinal tear has appeared, the patient may seek medical attention, and effective treatment of the tear may ensue. Unfortunately some patients do not seek attention, or, if they do, the symptoms may be disregarded. Indeed, in time the symptoms may become less, but after a period of a month or two (this period may vary between minutes and years), a black shadow is seen encroaching from the periph-

eral field. This may appear to wobble. If the detachment is above, the shadow encroaches from below and it may seem to improve spontaneously with bedrest, being at first better in the morning. Loss of central vision or visual blurring occurs when the fovea is involved by the detachment, or the visual axis is obstructed by a bullous detachment. Inspection of the fundus at this stage shows that fluid seeps through the retinal hole, raising up the surrounding retina like a blister in the paintwork of a car. A shallow detachment of the retina may be difficult to detect but the affected area tends to look slightly grey and, most importantly, the choroidal pattern can no longer be seen. The analogy is with a piece of wet tissue stuck against grained wood. If the tissue paper is raised slightly away from the wood, the grain is no longer visible. As the detachment increases, the affected area looks dark grey and corrugated and the retinal vessels look darker than in flat retina. The tear in the retina shines out red as one views the pigment epithelium and choroid through it.

Once a black shadow of this kind appears in front of the vision, the patient usually becomes alarmed and seeks immediate medical attention. Urgent admission to hospital and retina surgery are needed.

Traction Retinal Detachment

The retina may be pulled away by the contraction of fibrous bands in the vitreous, especially after perforating injuries of the eye. Photopsia and floaters are usually absent but a slowly progressive visual field defect is noticeable. The detached retina is usually concave and immobile. The symptoms and signs may be complicated by those of the original injury. Advanced proliferative diabetic retinopathy may be complicated by detachment of the retina when a contracting band either pulls away a piece of retina to produce a hole or simply tents up the retina by direct traction. When such a diabetic patient experiences sudden loss of vision in one eye, the most likely cause is vitreous haemorrhage or a superimposed rhegmatogenous retinal detachment.

Retinal Detachment Due to Tumours or Exudation

In such detachments there is no photopsia but floaters may occur from associated vitritis or vitreous haemorrhage. A visual field defect is usual. Exudative detachments are usually convex shaped and associated with shifting fluid.

A malignant melanoma of the choroid may present as a retinal detachment. Often the melanoma is evident as a black lump with an adjacent area of detached retina. If the retina is extensively detached over the tumour, the diagnosis may become difficult. It is important to avoid performing retinal surgery on such a case because of the risk of disseminating the tumour. Suspicion shouldbe raised by a balloon detachment without any visible tears, and the diagnosis may be confirmed by transilluminating the eye to reveal the tumour.

Exudative retinal detachments are not common. They are seen in patients with severe hypertensive retinopathy and toxaemia of pregnancy. Harada's disease is a symptom complex, which includes exudative uveitis with retinal detachment, patchy depigmentation of the skin, meningitis and deafness. Its cause is unknown. Exudative detachments do not require surgery but treatment of the underlying cause.

Management

Prophylaxis

Flat retinal tears can be sealed by means of light coagulation. A powerful light beam from a laser is directed at the surrounds of the tear (Figure 13.2). This produces blanching of the retina around the edges of the hole and, after some days, migration and proliferation of pigment cells occurs from the pigment epithelium into the neuroretina and the blanched area becomes pigmented. A bond is formed across the potential space and a retinal

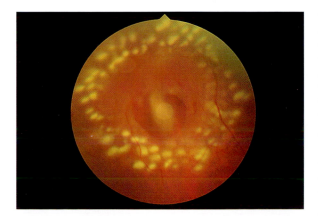

Fig. 13.2. Laser photocoagulation of retinal tear (with acknowledgement to Mr R. Gregson).

detachment is prevented. This procedure can be carried out, with the aid of a contact lens, in a few minutes. A wider and more diffuse area of chorioretinal bonding can be achieved by cryopexy, which entails freezing from the outside. Cryopexy is also necessary if the retinal hole is very peripheral. A cold probe is placed on the sclera over the site of the tear and an ice ball is allowed to form over the tear. A similar type of reaction (as occurs after photocoagulation) develops following this treatment, but it tends to be uncomfortable for the patient and local or general anaesthesia is required.

Retinal Surgery

In the early part of the twentieth century it was generally accepted that there was no known effective treatment for retinal detachment. It was realised that a period of bedrest resulted in flattening of the retina in many instances. This entailed a prolonged period of complete immobilisation with the patient lying flat with both eyes padded. This treatment can restore the sight but only temporarily because the retina re-detaches when the patient is mobilised. It was also very dangerous for the patient in view of the risk of venous thrombosis and pulmonary embolism. In the 1920s it began to be realised that effective treatment of retinal detachment depends on sealing the small holes in the retina (Figure 13.3). It was already known by then that the fluid under the retina could be drained off externally simply by puncturing the globe, but up till then no serious attempt had been made to associate this with some form of cautery to the site of the tear. Once it became apparent that cautery to the site of the tear combined with the release of subretinal fluid was effective, it also became evident that not all cases responded to this kind of treatment. It was almost as if the retina was too small for the eye in some cases, an idea, which led to the design of volume-reducing operations, which effectively made the volume of the globe smaller. This in turn led to the concept of mounting the tear on an inward protrusion of the sclera to prevent subsequent re-detachment.

Modern retinal surgery involves the sewing of small inert pieces of material, usually silicone rubber onto the outside of the sclera in such a way as to make a suitable indent at the site of the tear (Figure 13.4). This is preceded by cryopexy to the hole. It is often necessary to drain off the subretinal fluid and inject air or gas into the vitreous. In more difficult cases the eye may be encircled with a

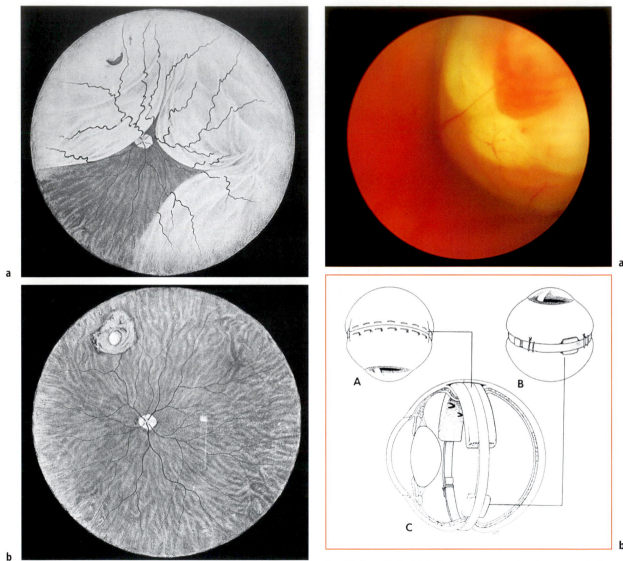

Fig. 13.3. Retinal detachment (a) before and (b) after treatment. (After Gonin).

Fig. 13.4.   **a** Retinal detachment surgery: retinal tear surrounded by cryopexy and covered by indent. **b** Retinal detachment surgery: indent and encirclement band (with acknowledgement to Professor D. Archer).

silicone strap to provide all-round support to a retina with extensive degenerative changes. In spite of the development of surgical techniques, some cases still provide difficulties. The retina can sometimes become so extensively torn that it folds up on itself and or the damaged retina may become fixed by the growth of a fine fibrous membrane across its inner or outer surface. Vitrectomy supplemented by a number of ingenious techniques has been developed in order to deal with such problems.

Prognosis

The retina can now be replaced by one operation in about 85% of cases. Of the successful cases, a proportion do not achieve a full restoration of their central vision, although usually the peripheral field recovers. The degree of recovery of central vision – that is, the ability to read the Snellen chart – depends largely on the duration of the detachment prior to surgery and whether the detachment was extensive enough to involve the macular region. Even when the retina has been detached for two years, it is still possible to restore useful navigational vision. When retinal surgery has failed, further surgery may be required and for a few patients a series of operations is necessary. If it is thought that more than one operation is going to be needed, then it is helpful to the patient if he or she is warned about this before the treatment is started.

Squint 14

The word "squint" refers to a failure of the visual axes to meet at the point of regard. For normal vision each eye must be focused on and lined up with the object of regard. The fact that we have two eyes positioned some 60 mm apart means that we can accumulate considerably more data about our environment than would be possible with one eye alone. This can best be exemplified by considering what happens when one eye is suddenly lost as the result of injury or disease. Apart from the obvious loss of visual field which necessitates turning the head to the blind side, the patient experiences impaired distance judgement. The skilled worker notices a deterioration in the ability to perform fine tasks and the elderly notice that they pour tea into the saucer rather than the cup. In time, depth perception may improve and the patient adapts to the defect to some extent; children may adapt to one eyed vision in a remarkable way. But it seems that modern civilised living does not have such great demands for binocular vision now that many tasks are carried out by machines. It is no coincidence that those animals whose survival depends on catching their food by means of accurate distance judgement have their eyes placed in front of their head, enabling the two eyes to be focused together on their prey.

Investigation of a normal human population reveals that although the eyes may be situated on the front of the face, they do not always work together, and it will be seen that there are a number of reasons why the mechanism may fail. The ability to use the eyes together is called binocular vision. It can be measured and graded by presenting each eye separately but simultaneously with a series of images. The instrument used to do this is called a synoptophore (Figure 14.1).

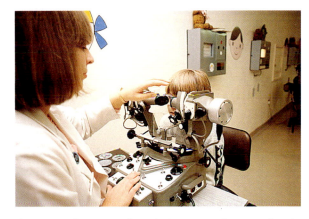

Fig. 14.1. The synoptophore. An instrument for measuring the angle of deviation of a squint and the ability of the eyes to work together.

1. *Simultaneous macular perception* is said to be present if the subject can see two dissimilar images which are presented simultaneously to each eye, for example, a triangle to one eye, a circle to the other.

2. *Fusion* is present if the subject can see two parts of a whole image as one whole when each half is presented to a separate eye. For example, a picture of a house to one eye, a picture of a chimney to the other, and the whole picture is maintained as one as the eyes converge. The range of fusion can be measured in degrees.

3. *Stereopsis*, the third grade of binocular vision, is present if, when slightly dissimilar views of an object are presented to each eye separately, a single three dimensional view of the whole is seen. Stereopsis itself can also be graded if very fine degrees of

impairment of binocular function need to be measured.

This ability of ours to put together the images from each eye and make a single picture in our minds seems to develop during the early years of life and furthermore its development seems to depend on visual input. Below the age of eight years any misalignment of the eyes which disturbs binocular vision may permanently damage this function.

If the alignment of the eyes is disturbed for any reason during childhood, the child may at first, as one might expect, notice double vision but very quickly learns to suppress the image from one eye, thereby eliminating the annoyance of diplopia at the expense of binocular vision. In fact most, but not all, children learn to suppress when using monocular instruments, switching the other eye on again when the instrument is not being used. Prolonged suppression seems to lead to a more permanent state of visual loss called amblyopia of disuse. The word "amblyopia" simply means blindness. Suppression is a temporary switching off of one eye when the other is in use, whereas amblyopia of disuse is a permanent impairment of vision, which could affect the career prospects of the patient. Amblyopia of disuse can also occur if the sight of one eye is defective as the result of opacities in the media, even though the alignment of the eyes has not been disturbed. Again this only occurs in children under the age of eight years. Covering one eye of a baby could lead to permanent impairment of the vision of that eye as well as impairment of the ability to use the eyes together. An adult may have one eye covered for many months or even years without suffering visual loss.

Before considering the causes and effects of squint in children and adults, it is necessary to know something of the different kinds of squint.

Types of Squint

In lay terms the "squint" can just mean screwing up the eyes, but here we are referring to a deviation of one eye from the line of sight. This may be present all the time or just when the patient is tired. It is important to notice whether the eye movements are normal. For example, if there is weakness of one lateral rectus muscle, the affected eye will not turn outwards and the angle of the squint will be much greater when looking to that side. Most childhood squints are not associated with weakness of one or more extraocular muscles so that the angle of the squint is the same in all directions of gaze. The deviation of the squint may be horizontal or sometimes vertical or the eyes may be convergent or divergent.

Squint in Childhood

During the first few weeks of life the eyes may seem to wander about aimlessly with limited ability to fix. Between the ages of two and six months, fixation becomes steadier even though the fovea is not fully developed, and by the age of six months convergence on a near object may be maintained for several seconds. Even at birth some degree of following movement of the eyes can be seen in response to a flashing light, but only the most gross squints can be diagnosed during these very early months of life. If the eyes are definitely squinting at the age of six months then urgent referral to an ophthalmologist is indicated. Prior to this or when there is some doubt, referral to an orthoptic screening service may be considered. These have been set up in many parts of the country. Orthoptists might be regarded as "physiotherapists of the eyes" and they are trained to examine the eye movements in great detail. We need to detect squints early in children for the following reasons:

- The squint may be caused by serious underlying intracranial or intraocular disease.
- The squint may result in amblyopia which is more effectively treated, the younger the child.
- The cosmetic effect of a squint is an important consideration.

Amblyopia of Disuse

A special mention is needed about this curious condition which accounts for unilateral impairment of vision in over 2% of the population. Any eye casualty officer is familiar with the patient with a foreign body on the cornea of one eye and the other eye being amblyopic ("How can I drive home with this patch on doctor?"). The words "lazy eye" are sometimes used but in lay terms this can also mean squint.

The eye suffering from amblyopia of disuse shows certain features:

- Impaired Snellen visual acuity but usually able to decipher vertical lines of letters better than horizontal ones.
- Normal fundus.

- Small residual squint or, if not, the affected eye relatively hypermetropic.
- An indefinite central scotoma which is difficult to assess by routine visual field testing.
- History of poor vision in one eye since childhood.

The diagnosis of amblyopia may be by exclusion but it must never be reached without a careful examination of the eyes. In recent years there has been a considerable research interest in this subject and there appear to be nerve conduction anomalies in the occipital cortex which can be induced by visual deprivation.

Causes of Squint in Childhood

- Refractive error – hypermetropia, myopia.
- Opaque media – corneal opacities, cataract, uveitis.
- Disease of retina or optic nerve – retinoblastoma, optic atrophy.
- Congenital or acquired weakness of extraocular muscles.
- Abnormalities of facial skeleton leading to displacement of extraocular muscles.

Refractive Error

In order to understand how refractive error can cause squint, one must first understand how the act of accommodation is linked to the act of convergence. That is to say, we must realise that when we focus upon an object, not only is each individual eye separately focused on it, but the eyes swivel together by the requisite amount to allow them both to view the object at once. A given amount of accommodation must therefore be associated with an equivalent amount of convergence. In hypermetropic subjects this relationship is disturbed. In order to overcome hypermetropia, the eyes must accommodate and sometimes this excessive focusing induces an excess of convergence hence causing a squint. This type of accommodative squint may be fully corrected by wearing spectacles; when the glasses are on the eyes are straight, when they are off one eye turns in. More often the squint is only partially accommodative and the squint is improved but not eliminated by wearing glasses. The convergent squint associated with hypermetropia is the commonest type of childhood squint.

Opaque Media

Congenital cataract can occasionally present as a squint. In a similar manner, a corneal opacity, as might result from herpes simplex keratitis or injury, may cause a squint to appear. A completely blind eye from whatever cause tends to converge if the blindness occurs in early childhood. Blindness of one eye in an adult tends to result in a divergent squint. This is sometimes a useful indicator of the age of onset of blindness.

Disease of the Retina or Optic Nerve

Such a possibility provides an important reason for the careful examination of the fundus in every case.

Congenital or Acquired Muscle Weakness

VIth, IIrd or IVth cranial nerve palsies are sometimes seen after head injuries and the surgeon must always bear in mind the possibility of a VIth or other cranial nerve palsy being associated with raised intracranial pressure. Myasthenia gravis is extremely rare in children but it may present as a squint. In some cases of squint there is a degree of facial asymmetry. These patients may also have "asymmetrical eyes', one being myopic or hypermetropic relative to the other. Sometimes there is no refractive error but there may be an asymmetry of the insertions of the extraocular muscles as a possible cause of squint. There is a group of conditions known as musculofascial anomalies in which there is marked limitation of the eye movements from birth in certain directions. They are accompanied by abnormal eye movements such as retraction of the globe and narrowing of the palpebral fissures on lateral gaze.

Overaction of muscles can cause a squint. This is seen in schoolchildren sometimes with a background of domestic or other stress. The eyes tend to overconverge and overaccommodate especially when being examined.

Diagnosis

History

When faced with a case of suspected squint there are certain aspects of the history, which may be very helpful in assisting with the diagnosis. It is often useful to ask who first noticed the squint. Sometimes a mother has been made anxious by a well-wishing neighbour or relative, and in these cases there may

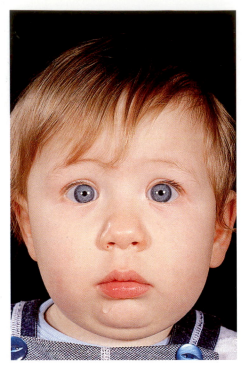

Fig. 14.2.   Pseudosquint. The configuration of the eyelids gives the appearance of a squint but the corneal reflexes show that this is not the case.

be no true squint but merely the appearance of one. The mother herself is usually the best witness. Unfortunately some children have a facial configuration which makes the eyes look as though they are deviating when they are not and it is essential that the student or general practitioner should be able to make this distinction in order to avoid sending unnecessary referrals to the local eye unit (Figure 14.2). Childhood squints often show a dominant pattern of inheritance and the family history provides a useful diagnostic indicator. From the point of view of prognosis it is useful to find out whether the squint is constant or intermittent and also the age of onset. A full ophthalmic history must be taken which should include the birth history and any illness which might have caused or initiated the problem.

Examination

While the history is being taken from the parents, one should be making an assessment of the child. If the child is obviously shy or nervous, a useful tech-

nique is to introduce something of interest to the child in the conversation with the parents. At this point it is important not to approach the child directly but to allow him or her to make an assessment of the doctor. It is quite impossible to examine an infant's eyes in a noisy room, thus the number of people present should be minimal and they should not be moving about. The room lighting should be dim enough to enable the light of a torch to be seen easily. The first important part of the examination is to shine a torch at the patient so that the reflection of the light can be seen on each cornea. The position of these corneal reflections is then noted carefully. The more mobile the child the less time there is to observe this. If there is a squint the reflections will be positioned asymmetrically in the pupil. If the patient has a left convergent squint, the reflection from the left cornea is displaced outwards towards the pupil margin. A rough assessment of the angle of the squint can be made at this stage by noting the abnormal position of the reflection. One of the difficulties experienced at this point is due to the continuous movement of the child's eyes, which make it difficult at first to know whether the light is being accurately fixated. By gently moving the torch slightly from side to side, it is usually possible to confirm that the child is looking, albeit momentarily, at the light.

Once the light reflections have been examined, the *cover test* can be performed. Once again the reflection of light from each eye is noted but this time one of the eyes is smartly covered, either with the back of the hand or a card. If the fixating eye is covered, a movement of the non-fixing eye to take up fixation may then be observed (Figure 14.3). After some practice it is possible to detect even very slight movements of this kind. The result of the test may be misleading if the non-fixing eye is too weak to take up fixation, and quite often, an assessment of the vision of the non-fixing eye can be made at this stage.

If, having performed this first stage of the cover test, no deviation can be detected then the cover can be quickly swapped from one eye to the other and any movement of the covered eye can be noted. That is to say, the latent deviation produced by covering one eye is spotted by noting the small recovery movement made by the previously covered eye. Finally the cover test must be repeated with the patient looking at a distant object. One type of squint in particular can be missed unless this is done. This is the divergent squint seen in young children, which is often only present when viewing

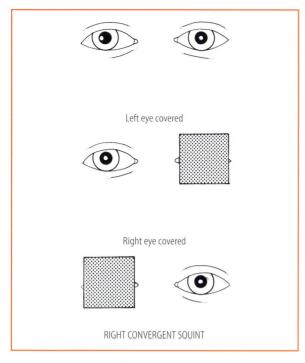

Left eye covered

Right eye covered

RIGHT CONVERGENT SQUINT

Fig. 14.3. The cover test.

distant objects. The parents may have noticed an obvious squint and yet testing by the doctor in the confines of a small room reveals nothing abnormal, with ensuing consternation all round.

After the cover test has been performed it is necessary to test the ocular movements to determine whether there is any muscle weakness. At this stage it is usual to instil a mydriatic and cycloplegic drop (e.g. cyclopentolate 1% or 0.5%) in order to obtain a measure of the refractive error, by retinoscopy, when the eyes are completely at rest. Next the optic fundi are examined.

In most instances the nature of the squint becomes apparent by this stage and further testing of the binocular function and more accurate measurement of the angle of the squint are carried out using the synoptophore.

Management of Squint in Childhood

Glasses

Any significant refractive error is corrected by the prescription of glasses. Sometimes the squint is completely straightened when glasses are worn but more often the control is partial, the glasses simply acting to reduce the angle of the squint. Glasses may be prescribed in a child as young as 6–9 months if really necessary. It is important that the parents have a full understanding of the need to wear glasses if adequate supervision is to be expected. When the spectacles are removed at bedtime, a previous squint may appear to become even worse and the parents should be warned about this possible rebound effect.

Orthoptic Follow-up

The orthoptic department forms an integral and important part of the modern eye unit. It is run and manned by orthoptists who carry out the careful measurement of visual acuity with and without glasses and the measurement of eye movements and binocular function. Once the patient has been seen for the initial visit, follow-up in the orthoptic department is arranged and the question of treatment by occlusion of the good eye has to be considered. By covering the good eye for a limited period, the sight of the amblyopic eye can be improved. The younger the child, the better are the chances of success. In older children, beyond the age of seven or eight years, not only is amblyopia more resistant to treatment, but the treatment itself can interfere seriously with schoolwork. The type and amount of occlusive treatment have to be planned and discussed with the parents. Sometimes atropine eye drops are used as an alternative to patching one eye. Orthoptic exercises may also be used in an attempt to strengthen binocular function.

Surgery

If the squint is not controlled by glasses, surgery should be considered. Some parents ask if an operation can be carried out as a substitute for wearing glasses. Unfortunately surgery to correct refractive error is not yet at a stage where it can be applied to children with squints. Squint surgery involves moving the muscle insertions or shortening the muscles and from the cosmetic point of view is highly effective. The adjustment of the muscles is measured in millimetres to correspond with the angle of the squint in degrees. Sometimes two or more operations are needed due to occasionally unpredictable results, but from the cosmetic point of view, nobody need suffer the indignity of a squint even though a series of operations may be needed. Once the eyes have been put straight or nearly straight by surgery, the functional result depends on the previous presence of good binocular vision and good vision in each eye.

Squint occurs in about 2% of the population and so it is a very common problem, but it is only a small proportion of these cases that eventually require surgery. The commonest type of squint in childhood is the accommodative convergent squint associated with hypermetropia and here surgery is indicated only when spectacles prove inadequate. Divergent squints are less common but more often require early surgery.

The aim of treatment for a child with squint is to make the eyes look straight, to make each eye see normally and to achieve good binocular vision. Unfortunately, all too often, the first one of these aims alone is achieved in spite of modern methods of treatment. The fault may lie partly in late referral or difficulty with patient co-operation but better methods of treatment are needed.

Squint in Adults

Adults who present with a squint have usually suffered defective action of one or more of the extraocular muscles. It is important to have a basic understanding of these muscles.

Anatomy of the Extraocular Muscles

These can be divided into three groups.

● *The horizontal recti*. The medial and lateral recti act as yoke muscles, like the reins of a horse. They rotate the eye about a vertical axis. The lateral rectus abducts the eye (turns it out) and the medial rectus adducts the eye (turns it in).

● *The vertical recti*. These act as vertical yoke muscles but they run diagonally from their origin at the apex of the orbit to be inserted 7 or 8 mm behind the limbus above and below the globe. The action of these muscles depends on the initial position of the eye. For example the primary action of the superior rectus is to elevate the abducted eye and the inferior rectus depresses the abducted eye. The secondary action of the superior rectus is to adduct and intort the adducted eye; the inferior rectus adducts and extorts the adducted eye. Intorsion and extorsion refer to rotation about an antero-posterior axis through the globe. The important thing to realise is that the action of these muscles depends on the position of the eye (Figure 14.4).

● *The obliques*. These are also vertical yoke muscles but they run on a different line to the vertical recti. The superior oblique depresses the adducted eye (makes the eye go down when it is turned in) and the inferior oblique elevates the adducted eye.

When a patient has a IVth cranial nerve palsy on the right side, the right eye can no longer look down when it is turned in due to the defective action of the superior oblique muscle. Double vision is experienced which is maximal (i.e. widest displacement of images) when looking down to the left.

When a patient has a VIth cranial nerve palsy on the right side, the right eye can no longer abduct or turn outwards. A right convergent squint is seen and the patient experiences double vision worse when

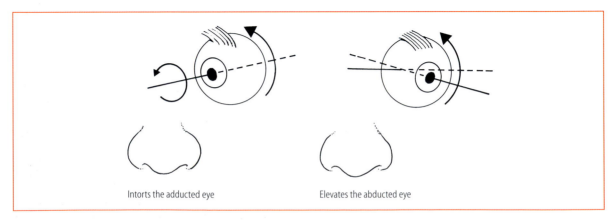

Intorts the adducted eye   Elevates the abducted eye

Fig. 14.4. Primary and secondary actions of the superior rectus muscle.

looking to the right. There may be a head turn to the right.

When a patient has a IIIrd cranial nerve palsy on the right side, the right eye is turned down and to the right and, if the palsy is complete, the upper lid droops and the pupil is dilated. Movement of the eye is very limited.

Causes of Adult Squint

Adults who *present* with a squint usually have a well-defined ocular muscle palsy. This may be due to a pathological process at any point from the brain, through the nerve to the muscle. These will be discussed elsewhere but two important causes are disseminated sclerosis in the younger age groups and hypertensive vascular disease in older patients. Diabetes is another important cause that must be excluded in all age groups.

Some adult squints prove to be concomitant squints neglected from childhood. Sometimes a latent squint, which has been well controlled throughout childhood, breaks down in adult life.

In adult life a blind eye tends to turn outwards and a divergent squint may be due solely to impaired vision in one eye.

Diagnosis

In contrast to the situation with children, who usually present with concomitant squint associated with hypermetropia, the sudden onset of a squint in adult life is extremely disabling because of intractable double vision. The double vision is less apparent when the lesion is more central, involving the level of the cranial nerve nucleus or above. In the latter case, the patient tends to complain more of blurred vision and confusion.

A carefully taken history may reveal the diagnosis. First it is necessary to ensure that the double vision is only present with both eyes open and then the patient can be questioned about the position of the second image and whether the separation of the images is maximal in any particular direction of gaze. The duration and constant or intermittent nature of the squint must be determined as must the history of any associated disease, past or present.

Once the history has been obtained, the nature of the squint can be investigated by the cover test and measured by the Maddox wing and Maddox rod. An accurate record of the impaired muscle action can be recorded on the Hess screen.

Maddox Wing

This ingenious, but simple, device is held in the patient's hand. By looking through the eyepieces, one eye is made to look at an arrow and the other eye at a row of numbers. If the eyes are straight, the arrow points at zero, and if not, the arrow indicates the angle of the squint.

Maddox Rod

The Maddox wing measures the deviation at reading distance and the Maddox rod is a similar device to measure the deviation when viewing a distant object. A special optical glass is placed in front of one eye, which turns the image of a light source into a line image. One eye, therefore, views the point source of light and the other a line, and the separation of these two images can be measured on a scale.

Hess Screen

Here the eyes are dissociated by using either coloured filters or a mirror. The system is arranged so that a screen is viewed with one eye and the end of a pointer with the other. The patient is told to place the pointer on various points on the screen. If the eyes are not straight the pointer is placed away from the correct position. A map of the incorrect positions is made (Figure 14.5). The shape of the map is diagnostic of particular ocular muscle problems and serial records can be very helpful in assessing progress.

Treatment

Many cases of adult squint recover spontaneously within a period of 3–6 months. Once the cause of the squint has been investigated the immediate treatment entails eliminating the diplopia by occluding one or other eye. This may be conveniently achieved by applying adhesive tape to the spectacle lens. If the angle of the squint is sufficiently small, it may be possible to regain binocular vision by means of a prism. Fresnel prisms are thin and flexible and can be simply stuck on the spectacle lens as a temporary measure during the recovery period. When the squint shows no sign of recovery over a period of nine months or more, then surgery is usually required to restore binocular vision. Before applying these principles of management it is essential to treat the underlying cause of the squint. It would be a serious error to treat diplopia due to raised

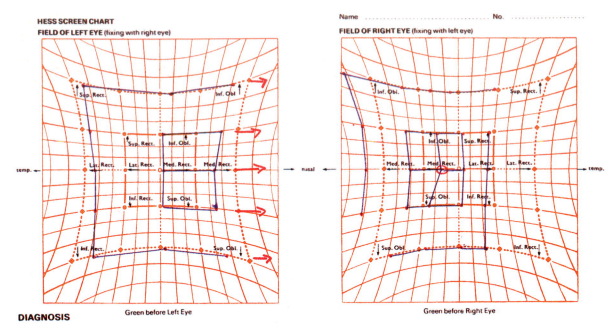

Fig. 14.5. Hess chart depicting a right lateral rectus palsy.

Ocular Muscle Imbalance

intracranial pressure by means of prisms without instituting a full neurological investigation, just as it would not help the patient with myasthenia gravis to undergo squint surgery before medical treatment has been started.

Mild latent squints may sometimes go undetected until a period of stress or perhaps excessive reading precipitates symptoms of eyestrain and headache. The effort to maintain both eyes in line causes the symptoms. The latent deviation may be inwards or outwards but because most people's eyes tend to assume a slightly divergent position when com-

pletely at rest, a degree of latent divergence (exophoria) is almost the rule and of no significance. Vertical muscle imbalance is less well tolerated and even a slight deviation may cause symptoms. Small but significant degrees of vertical muscle imbalance are seen in otherwise normal individuals who show a marked difference in refractive error between the two eyes or in those with facial asymmetry. The provision of a small prism incorporated into the spectacle lenses of such patients may produce dramatic relief, but we must always remember that the appearance of an ocular muscle imbalance may be the first indication of more serious disease. A small vertical deviation may be the first sign of a tumour of the lacrimal gland or thyrotoxic eye disease and a wide range of investigations may be needed before one can be satisfied with the excellent results of symptomatic treatment.

Tumours of the Eye and Adnexae 15

In this chapter the more important ocular tumours will be considered. There are a considerable number of other rare tumours and the interested student should refer to one of the more specialised and comprehensive textbooks of ophthalmology for further reading.

The Globe

Expanding tumours in the eye present diagnostic problems because it is not usually possible to biopsy them.

Choroidal Melanoma

The commonest intraocular tumour is the malignant melanoma of the choroid. It is the commonest primary intraocular tumour in adults. It is extremely rare in black people. In white people the average age of patients with choroidal melanoma is 50 years and the incidence rises at 70 years. However, it is important to appreciate that no age is exempt since choroidal melanomas have been reported in children as young as three years old. It differs from melanoma of the skin in that it grows more slowly and metastasises late. At first it is seen as a raised pigmented oval area which may be anywhere in the fundus (Figure 15.1). It is usually brown in colour although it may be amelanotic (or greyish). As the tumour enlarges there may be an associated exudative retinal detachment or, less often, secondary glaucoma. Other associated features may include choroidal haemorrhage and serial photography may be needed to confirm the growth. The usual presentation is with decreased vision or a visual field defect. Diagnosis is confirmed with careful clinical

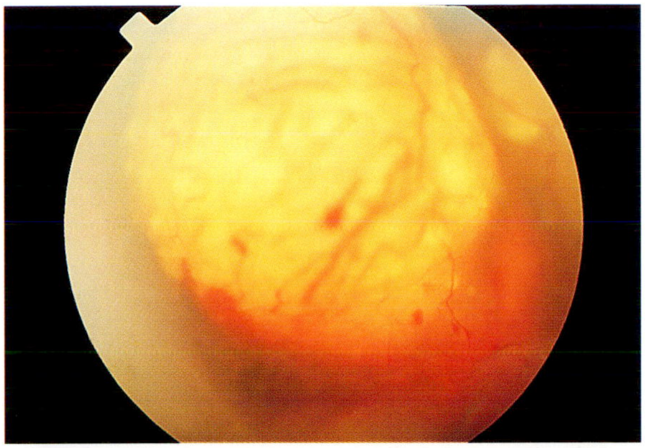

a

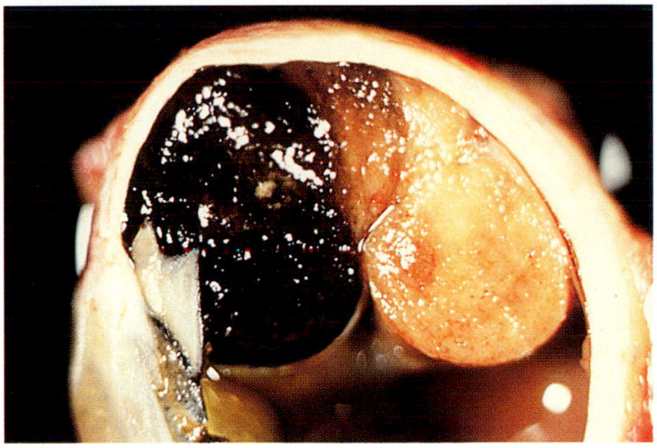

b

Fig. 15.1. Choroidal melanoma poorly pigmented (amelanotic) melanoma a) fundus photograph. b) Bisected eye showing pigmented and nonpigmented portions of melanoma in same eye (with acknowledgement to Mr A. Foss).

examination including indirect ophthalmoscopy and slit-lamp biomicroscopy (contact lens or volk lens examination), fluorescein angiography and ultrasonography. Metastases have to be excluded by liver function tests, liver ultrasound and chest X-rays.

The differential diagnosis of choroidal melanoma includes retinal detachment, metastatic choroidal tumours, exudative macular degeneration, choroidal naevi, haemangioma or choroidal effusions. The appearance of metastases may be delayed for several years and may occur even if the eye has been removed. Most cases are still treated by removal of the eye, but radiotherapy and local removal or resection of the tumour have been advocated and justified by the ultimate poor prognosis following enucleation (surgical excision of the eye). Untreated, the tumour may extend into the orbit and provide an unpleasant problem for the patient.

Retinoblastoma

This is a rare tumour of childhood which arises not from the choroid but, as its name suggests, from the retina. It is, however, the commonest primary intraocular tumour in children. It shows certain rather strange and unusual features. It is not usually present from birth, but occurs most frequently in infancy to three years (although it can occur in older patients); it is usually inherited as an autosomal dominant or may be sporadic, and in one-third of cases appears in both eyes. A change in chromosome 13 is found in the inherited cases. Initially it may be seen in an individual, suspected on account of the family history, as small white, raised mass. Examination under anaesthesia is essential in such cases because the tumour may be in the extreme periphery of the fundus. A larger tumour may present as a white mass in the pupil ("leucocoria") and such an appearance in infancy demands immediate referral to an ophthalmologist (Figure 15.2). Other presenting features include strabismus, secondary glaucoma, proptosis or inflammatory signs. Extension tends to occur locally up the optic nerve and enucleation is often life saving. CT scanning and ultrasound may show a calcified intraocular mass. Smaller tumours can be treated effectively by radiotherapy and many patients now survive into adult life. Genetic counselling is essential for these patients in order to prevent the increasing incidence of the tumours, which will result from effective medical treatment.

Melanoma of the Iris

This rare pigmented iris tumour causes distortion of the pupil, which may be a warning sign. Other features which may point to the diagnosis are localised lens opacity, neovascularisation and elevation of

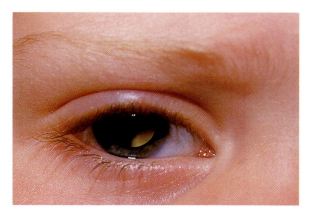

Fig. 15.2.   Retinoblastoma: leucocoria.

intraocular pressure. It is extremely slow growing and probably much less malignant than choroidal melanomas. It usually presents as a solitary iris nodule, which may or may not be pigmented.

The Eyelids

Benign Tumours

Meibomian Cysts (Chalazion)

This is the commonest eyelid lump in all ages. It is due to blockage of the meibomian gland orifice such that the secretions accumulate. A granulomatous inflammation is set up which results in a painless, round, firm slowly growing lump in the tarsal plate (Figure 15.3). The cyst may become infected when it becomes red, hot and painful.

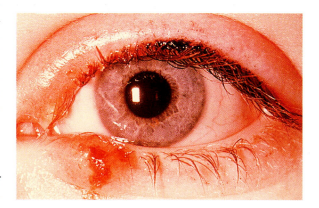

Fig. 15.3.   Chalazion.

Molluscum Contagiosum

This is viral infection most commonly seen in children. The lesions consist of several pale, waxy, umbilicated nodules on the eyelids and face. Similar lesions may be located on the trunk. The eyelid lesions shed viral particles, which produce a chronic conjunctivitis and less often superficial keratitis. The lesions may disappear in about six months, but may need curettage or cautery.

Papilloma

This is the name used to describe a rather common virus induced nodule or filiform wart often seen on the lid margin.

Seborrhoeic Keratosis

This is common in the elderly and consists of slow growing sessile, greasy lesions of the eyelid. They are usually brown and friable.

Senile keratosis consists of multiple, flat, scaly lesions, which may occasionally undergo transformation into a squamous cell carcinoma.

Xanthelasma

These are slightly elevated lesions consisting of lipid deposits usually on the medial aspect of the eyelids. They may be associated with hyperlipidaemia especially in the younger patient.

Keratoacanthoma

This is an example of a lesion, which grows rapidly, too rapidly for a neoplasm, over a period of a few weeks and then resolves spontaneously (Figure 15.4).

It usually starts as a red papule, which grows quickly into a nodule with a keratin filled crater. The lesion may resemble a basal cell carcinoma. Small lumps on the eyelids should be removed and biopsied. Larger lumps may be biopsied by taking a small segment from then prior to total excision if this proves necessary. Special care should be taken with the excision of any lesion on the eyelid in view of the risk of causing distortion of the lid margin or exposure keratitis.

Kaposi Sarcoma

This is a well-known association with acquired immune deficiency syndrome (AIDS). The lesions consist of purple nodules on the eyelid and similar lesions in the lower conjunctival fornix composed of proliferating endothelial and spindle shape cells. Inflammatory cells may also be present with vascular channels without endothelial cell lining.

Benign Pigmented Lesions of the Conjunctiva

Conjunctival epithelial melanosis occurs in approximately 90% of black and 10% of white people, and is noticeable in early life. The lesions are flat, brownish patches scattered throughout the conjunctiva, but may be more noticeable at the limbus (Figure 15.5). Usually they do not grow.

Other pigmented lesions require closer attention and specialist evaluation.

Pingueculum

This is a common mass lesion of the conjunctiva. It is seen as a yellowish nodule usually on the

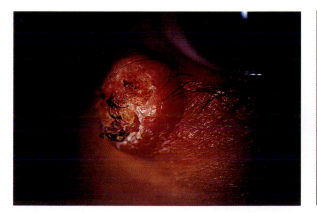

Fig. 15.4. Keratoacanthoma (with acknowledgement to Mr A. Sadiq).

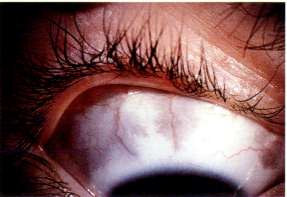

Fig. 15.5. Conjunctival melanosis.

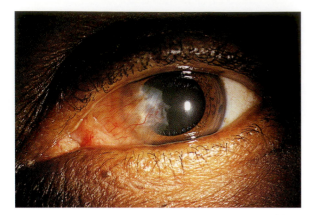

Fig. 15.6. Pterygium.

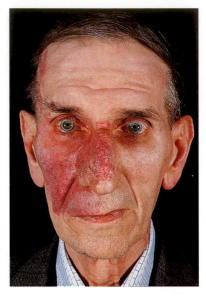

Fig. 15.7. Port wine stain (naevus flammeus).

medial interpalpebral fissure. It is a fibrovascular degeneration and is seen in all climates.

Pterygium

This is a growth of abnormal fibrovascular tissue extending from the conjunctiva over the cornea (Figure 15.6). It is thought to be due to chronic irritation from dust and solar radiation. It is more common in hot climates and individuals that work out of doors. Recurrent inflammation of the pterygium is often self-limiting but responds to a short course of topical steroids. If it extends over the visual axis of the cornea it may cause visual impairment. Surgical excision may be required.

Benign Vascular Tumours of the Eyelids

These fall into three types:

● *Capillary haemangioma of the newborn (strawberry naevus).* This is seen frequently usually before the age of six months, and nearly all examples regress spontaneously usually in few months and by the age of five years. Tumours appear as red, slightly raised marks on the skin. Even very extensive tumours of this kind can show a dramatic improvement over several years and conservative management is usually indicated unless the tumour is associated with a fold of skin, which occludes the eye. Larger tumours may produce orbital enlargement. The possibility of amblyopia of disuse and anisometropia must always be borne in mind.

● *Cavernous haemangioma.* These tumours lie more deeply in the skin and appear as a bluish swelling in the lid which expands when the child cries. These lesions may also disappear spontaneously or, if persistent, they may be treated by freezing.

● *Telangiectatic haemangioma.* Also known as the port wine stain or naevus flammeus, this tumour tends to be distributed over the area supplied by one or more of the branches of the Vth cranial nerve and usually remains throughout life as a dark red discoloration in the skin (Figure 15.7). The importance of this particular appearance is its association with secondary glaucoma and haemangioma of the meninges. The latter produces calcification and a characteristic X-ray appearance. The combination of lesions is known as the Sturge–Weber syndrome. There may be hypertrophy of the affected area of the face leading to asymmetry.

Malignant Tumours of the Eyelids

Basal Cell Carcinoma

This is the commonest malignant tumour of the eyelids in adults. It commonly involves the lower lid and medial canthus. The tumour begins as a small insignificant nodule, which turns into a small crater-like lesion with a slightly raised edge (Figure 15.8). At this stage it is a simple matter to remove the lesion and confirm the diagnosis by biopsy, but if left the tumour tends to spread and the prognosis becomes worse once the underlying bone is invaded

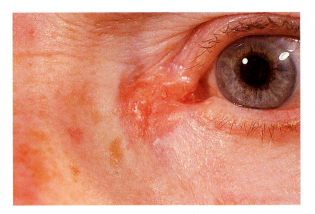

Fig. 15.8. Early basal cell carcinoma of medial canthus.

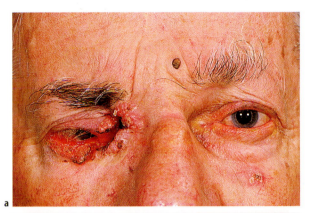

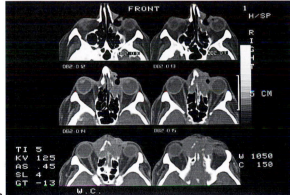

Fig. 15.9. Extensive basal cell carcinoma involving the orbit and extending across the nose to the opposite side. **a** Clinical photograph; **b** computerised tomography scan.

(Figure 15.9). This is the case with canthal tumours. Extensive neglected basal cell carcinomata are treated palliatively by radiotherapy or extensive surgery. They very rarely metastasise.

Squamous Cell Carcinoma

It is the second most common malignant eyelid lesion. This tumour may initially resemble the basal cell carcinoma although the edges are usually not rolled. Spread tends to occur to the local lymph nodes, (preauricular for the upper lid and submandibular for the lower lid), and the tumour is liable to metastasise.

Sebaceous Gland Carcinoma

These uncommon tumours arise from meibomian glands. It appears as a discrete, firm nodule, which often presents as a "recurrent chalazion". Delayed diagnosis increases mortality significantly.

Melanoma of the Eyelid and Conjunctiva

Malignant melanoma of the eyelids is similar to malignant melanoma elsewhere, appearing as a raised often shiny black lump. It metastasises at a very early stage and the prognosis does not seem to be altered by excision. Malignant melanomata may also occur on the conjunctiva (Figure 15.10) but they should not be confused with the relatively common benign conjunctival naevus. The latter is a slightly raised pigment-stippled lesion often seen at the limbus on the temporal side. Closer examination with the hand lens or microscope reveals one or two minute cysts. It is generally accepted that these lesions should be excised if they become irritable or sometimes simply on cosmetic grounds, but they rarely become malignant.

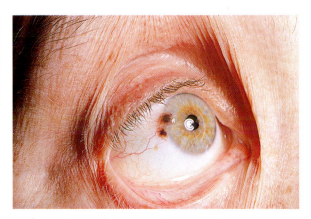

Fig. 15.10. Melanoma of conjunctiva.

Table 15.1.   Primary orbital tumours

Vascular	Capillary haemangioma
	Cavernous haemangioma
	Lymphangioma
Neural	Optic nerve glioma
	Meningioma
	Neurofibromatoma
Lacrimal gland	
Lymphorpoliferative	
Rhabdomyosarcoma	
Histiocytosis	

The Orbit (see Table 15.1)

Lacrimal Gland and Sac Tumours

Lacrimal gland tumours may either be inflammatory, mixed cell tumours or adenocarcinomas. They present with proptosis or mass in the outer part of the eyelid superotemporal orbit. Lacrimal sac tumours are less common and present with sac swelling. Benign lesions and infections need to be excluded.

Dermoid Cyst

This cystic swelling is usually seen at the level of the eyebrow in the upper outer part of the orbit. It is smooth and fluctuant and often fixed to bone. Sometimes a deeper part of the cyst may occupy a cavity in the bone and a CT scan is advisable when this is suspected. Excision on cosmetic grounds and for diagnosis is usually indicated.

Cavernous Haemangioma

This is the commonest primary neoplasm of the orbit in adults. It is benign. It is unusual for surgery to be necessary in such cases. It is usually located within the muscle cone, and gives rise to axial proptosis.

Glioma of the Optic Nerve

This rare tumour causes progressive proptosis and optic atrophy but it may be very slow growing. There is an association with von Recklinghausen's disease, and the presence of pigmented patches in the skin should make one suspect this.

Rhabdomyosarcoma

This rare but highly malignant orbital tumour is seen in children. Its growth is so rapid that it may be misdiagnosed as orbital cellulitis. If a correct diagnosis is made at an early stage, there is some hope of reaching a cure by combining radiotherapy and chemotherapy. The tumour is thought to arise from striated muscle and the histological diagnosis is confirmed by finding striation in the tumour cells. It is usually located in the superonasal orbit.

Metastatic Tumours and Tumours from Neighbouring Sites

A wide variety of tumours may invade the orbit and produce proptosis and often diplopia. Lymphoma is one example. It may present as an isolated lesion or in association with Hodgkin's disease or leukaemia. Examples of local spread from adjacent structures include carcinoma of the nasopharynx, carcinoma of the lacrimal gland and meningioma. In children orbital metastases arise most commonly from neuroblastoma and Ewing's sarcoma. In the adult the commonest primary sites are bronchus, breast, prostate and kidneys.

"Pseudotumour"

This is an inflammatory swelling in the orbit of unknown cause, which may present with pain, proptosis and diplopia. A mass may be palpable in the orbit and biopsy reveals non-specific inflammatory tissue consisting mainly of lymphocytes. Diagnosis may eventually be made by exclusion of other causes of proptosis. In severe cases a course of systemic steroids and or radiotherapy is usually very effective

Exophthalmos and Proptosis

Both these terms mean forward protrusion of the eyes but traditionally exophthalmos refers to the bilateral globe protrusion in thyroid disease. Proptosis refers to unilateral forward displacement of the globe from whatever cause. In practice the terms tend to be used rather loosely and are now almost synonymous (Figure 15.11).

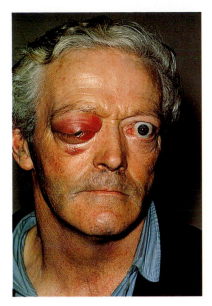

Fig. 15.11.   Proptosis: dysthyroid disease.

achieved from the history, examination and tests of thyroid function.

- *Infection*. Orbital cellulitis, usually from neighbouring sinuses, requires urgent otorhinological opinion.
- *Trauma*. Proptosis can occur as a result of retro-orbital haemorrhage. Diagnosis should be possible from the patient's history.
- *Haemangioma*. This may expand after bending down or crying. Ultrasound and CT scanning may confirm the diagnosis. Occasionally angiography, may be required
- *Pseudotumour*. Biopsy should be carried out if possible, and other causes excluded.
- *Mucocele of sinuses*. Diagnose by X-ray or CT scan.
- *Lymphoproliferative disease*. A biopsy, full blood count and sternal marrow puncture should be carried out.
- *Others*. There are a large number of possible but rare causes of proptosis.

Causes of Proptosis (see Table 15.2)

When one eye seems to bulge forward the doctor may have a serious problem on his or her hands and the following likely causes should be considered:

- *Pseudoproptosis*. An apparent bulging forward of the eye occurs if the eye is too big, as in unilateral high myopia or if the other eye is sunken following a blow-out fracture of the maxilla (orbital floor). These need to be distinguished from a true proptosis.
- *Thyrotoxicosis*. This is the commonest cause of unilateral or bilateral proptosis; diagnosis is

Table 15.2.   Causes of proptosis

- Endocrine
- Vascular abnormalities
- Inflammatory disorders
- Primary orbital tumours
- Metastases

Assessment of Proptosis

In the clinic, proptosis is best assessed by standing behind the seated patient and asking him or her to look down. The position of each globe in relation to the lids and face can be best seen by this means. Proptosis can be measured by means of an exophthalmometer. A number of such instruments are on the market and they depend on measuring the distance from the rim of the outer margin of the orbit to the level of the anterior part of the cornea. These measurements are not always very accurate (especially for the novice) but best results are achieved by ensuring that they are made by the same person on each occasion for a given patient.

Once thyroid disease and trauma have been excluded, the patient would require further investigations including systemic examination, full blood picture, orbital ultrasound, CT scan, MRI scan, possibly carotid angiography and sometimes orbital biopsy.

Ocular Trauma

The fact that injuries to the eye and its surrounding region demand special attention and create great concern for patient and doctor is self-evident when the eye alone is involved, but when other life-threatening injuries are present the eye injury, seeming slight at the time, may be overlooked. Sometimes the eyelids may be so swollen that it is difficult to examine the eyes and a serious perforating injury may be obscured. When other injuries are present and an anaesthetic is needed, it is essential that the eyes are examined carefully, if possible under the same anaesthetic. As in the case of injuries elsewhere, those to the eye demand urgent and immediate treatment, and neglect can result in tragedy even though the problem may have at first seemed very slight.

Injuries to the Globe

Contusion

The eye casualty officer comes to recognise a familiar pattern of contusion, the effect of squash-ball injuries and blows from flying objects in industry or after criminal assault. Injuries from industrial causes have now become quite uncommon thanks to better control by means of protective clothing and proper guarding of machinery. Sporting injuries have as a result become more evident although here also increasing public concern has led some improvement. Notable instances of good control are the use of protective guards in ice hockey and cricket. The surrounding orbital margin provides good protection to the eyes from footballs and even tennis and cricket balls but the rare golf ball contusion injury usually leads to loss of the sight of the eye.

Squash balls and especially shuttlecocks have earned a bad reputation for inflicting contusion injuries and, from the economic point of view, leading to loss of time at work and hospital expenses.

The extent of damage to the eye from contusion depends on whether it has been possible to close the eyelids in time before the moment of impact. If the lids have been closed, bruising and swelling of the eyelids is marked and the injury to the eye may be minimal. It must be remembered though that this is not an infallible rule and the eyes themselves must always be carefully examined, even when there is extreme swelling of the lids. It is always possible to examine an eye, if necessary using an eye speculum under general anaesthesia. In the primary care situation one must be very careful not to apply more than gentle pressure to the eyelids in case the globe of the eye has been perforated and when there is doubt referral to the eye department is advisable. The important clinical features of contusion injury are best considered by looking at the anatomical parts of the eye.

Cornea

The commonest injury to the cornea is from the corneal foreign body and this has already been described in Chapter 5. Almost as common is the corneal abrasion. It is odd how this is so often caused by the edge of a newspaper, a comb or a child's fingernail. Abrasions from the leaves of plants or twigs need special attention because of the type of infection that can occur, but any abrasion can lead to the condition known as recurrent abrasion. Here the patient experiences a sharp pain in the eye in the early morning usually on waking. It is thought that the lid margin adheres to the area of weakened cornea during sleep. The condition can occur months or even years after the original injury. The diagnosis is easily missed if the patient has forgotten about the original injury and if the cornea is not examined carefully with the slit-lamp microscope. This problem of recurrence is a reason to treat these abrasions with some care and to provide the patient with a lubricating ointment to be used for some time after the original injury has healed. Sometimes recurrent abrasion is due to a rare inherited disorder of the corneal epithelium.

When a patient presents with a corneal abrasion, the eyelids are often swollen perhaps from rubbing and the distress and agitation can be considerable. Examination may be impossible without first instilling a drop of local anaesthetic. These drops should never be continued as treatment because they would seriously delay the healing of the cornea.

Anterior Chamber

A small bleed into the anterior chamber of the eye is seen as a fluid level of blood inferiorly ("hyphaema"). This is a sign of potential problems because of the risk of secondary bleeding after two or three days. This risk is especially serious in children and the complication can lead to secondary glaucoma and at worst the loss of the eye. The parents need to be warned about this if there is a hyphaema.

Iris

When confronted by a flying missile, the normal reaction is to attempt to close the eyelids and to rotate the eyes upwards. This is the reason why the commonest point of impact is the lower temporal part of the eye and it is in this region of the iris that one is most likely to see peripheral iris tears ("iridodialysis").

When the eye is compressed the iris periphery is torn at its root, leaving a crescentic gap which looks black, but through which the fundus and red reflex can be observed. Such an injury also provides an excellent view of the peripheral part of the lens and the zonular ligament (Figure 16.1).

Contusion may result not in a tear of the iris root, but in a tangential splitting of the iris and ciliary body from the sclera producing recession of the angle of the anterior chamber; the appearance is often associated with secondary glaucoma and is identified using the special contact lens known as the gonioscope.

A sudden impact on the eye may also produce microscopic radial tears in the pupillary sphincter of the iris. This may be a subtle microscopic sign of

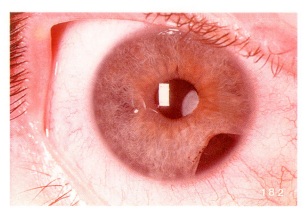

Fig. 16.1. Iridodialysis or splitting of the iris root in lower temporal quadrant. A sure sign of previous contusion.

previous injury when no other signs are present, or the damage may be more severe resulting in persistent dilatation of the pupil (traumatic mydriasis). Unless the eye is examined this widening of the pupil after injury can be mistaken for a third cranial nerve palsy.

Lens

Any severe contusion of the eye is liable to cause cataract, but the lens may not become opaque for many years after the injury. The lens may also become subluxated (slightly displaced due to partial rupture of the zonular ligament) or even dislocated either anteriorly or posteriorly.

Vitreous

The vitreous may become displaced after a contusion injury if it has not already undergone this change as part of the normal ageing process. The patient may be aware of something floating in front of the vision. More extensive floating black spots can indicate a vitreous haemorrhage. Although such haemorrhages usually clear completely in time they tend to accompany more serious damage to the retina which may only be fully revealed once clearing has taken place.

Retina

Bruising and oedema of the retina are seen as grey areas with scattered haemorrhages. The macular region is susceptible to oedema after contusion injuries causing permanent damage to the reading vision. Just as tears can occur to the peripheral iris,

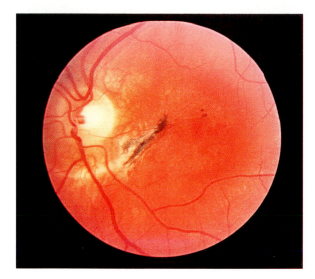

Fig. 16.2.   Healed choroidal tear. Another sign of previous injury.

so a similar problem is seen in the peripheral retina. These crescentic retinal dialyses are also most common in the lower temporal quadrant and their importance lies in the fact that they may lead to a detachment of the retina unless the tear is sealed by laser treatment. Any significant contusion injury of the eye requires a careful inspection of the peripheral retina.

Choroid

Tears in the choroid following contusion have a characteristic appearance. They are concentric with the disc and are seen as white crescents where the sclera is exposed. When near the macula, there is usually permanent damage to the central vision (Figure 16.2).

Optic Nerve

A variable degree of optic atrophy may become apparent a few weeks after a contusion injury. Blunt injuries to the eye may cause bleeding into the optic nerve sheath, and this can result in complete loss of vision on the affected side, the blindness being permanent. Attempts have been made to relieve the situation by emergency decompression of the optic nerve.

Perforation

As soon as the globe of the eye is penetrated there is a serious risk of infection. The vitreous is an ex-

cellent culture medium and in the pre-antibiotic era eyes were totally lost within two or three days as a result of this. *A perforating wound of the eye must therefore be considered a surgical emergency.* Perforating injuries are seen in children from scissor blades, screwdrivers, darts and other more bizarre objects. In adults there has been a dramatic fall in the incidence of such injuries since the introduction of compulsory seat belts but "do-it-yourself" accidents and assaults still take their toll. Following such an injury it is important to consider the possibility of an intraocular foreign body especially when there is a history of using a hammer and chisel.

The outcome of a perforating injury is dependent on the depth of penetration and the care with which the wound is cleaned and sutured. If the cornea alone is damaged, excellent results may be obtained by careful suturing under general anaesthesia using the operating microscope. If the lens has been damaged, early cataract surgery may be needed and deeper penetration may result in the need for retinal detachment surgery.

On admission or in the casualty department, the patient is given tetanus prophylaxis and both systemic and local antibiotics. If early surgery under general anaesthesia is likely to be needed then it is better for the patient not to eat or drink to avoid delays in hospital. If it becomes clear that the injury is a serious one, it is better to warn the patient at an early stage about the possible risk of losing the sight of the eye or even the need to replace it with an artificial one.

Intraocular Foreign Body

Metallic foreign bodies tend to enter the eyes of those who operate high-speed grinders without goggles or those using a hammer and chisel on metal without protection. These injuries may seem slight at first and sometimes the patient does not attach much importance to it. *Any such eye injury with this occupational history warrants an X-ray of the eye.* When ferrous metals remain in the eye they may cause immediate infection, or at a later date the deposition of ferrous salts in a process known as siderosis. This may eventually lead to blindness of the eye. Other metals also tend to give reactions, and for this reason the metallic fragment should be removed (Figure 16.3). This is achieved either by using intravitreous forceps under microscopic control or using a magnet. The exact surgical technique is planned beforehand once the foreign body has been accurately localised in the eye. Airgun

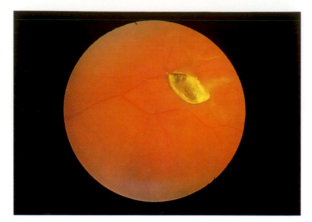

Fig. 16.3.   A small metallic foreign body lying on the retina.

pellets cause particularly severe eye injuries and the eye is often lost because of the extensive disruption at the time of the injury. Some intraocular foreign bodies such as glass particles or some alloys may be tolerated quite well and a decision may have to be made as to whether observation is preferable in the first instance. This especially applies when the sight of the eye remains good. When a foreign body is found lying deeply in the cornea, its removal may result in loss of aqueous and collapse of the anterior chamber. It is prudent to arrange that removal should be done under full sterile conditions in the operating theatre where the corneal wound can be sutured if necessary.

Sympathetic Ophthalmia

This rare complication of perforation is more common in children. The injured eye remains markedly inflamed and the wound may have been cleaned inadequately or too late. Over a period of two weeks to several months or even years a particular type of inflammatory response begins in the uvea and subsequently a similar reaction occurs in the other eye. The inflammation in both eyes can be so severe as to cause blindness. The condition does however respond well to steroid treatment and is extremely rare. Occasionally one sees patients who have an artificial eye complaining of transient blurring of the vision of their remaining eye. They need to be examined carefully for signs of uveitis.

Injuries to the Eyelids

Loss or destruction of eyelid tissue should always be treated as a threat to vision. The upper lid especially is important in this respect. The immediate concern is to ensure that the cornea is properly covered when the eyelids are closed. If more than one-third of the margin of the upper lid is lost, this must be replaced by grafting from the lower lid. When less than one-third is missing, the gaping wound can usually be closed directly. Up to one-third of the lower lid can also be closed by direct suturing. When more than this is lost or when it has been transferred to the upper lid, a slide of tissue from the lateral canthus can be effected, combined if necessary with a rotating cheek flap.

One of the most important features of the repair of lid injuries is the method of suturing. If the lid margin is involved, the repair should be made using the operating microscope and the fine suture material available in an eye department. An untidy repair can result in a permanently watering eye due to kinking of the eyelid. This interferes with the proper moistening of the cornea during blinking or when asleep. Special attention must be paid when the medial part of the eyelid has been torn and if this involves the lacrimal canaliculus. Again unless repair is carried out using an accurate technique under general anaesthesia in theatre then the risk of a permanently watering eye is increased.

Contusion of the eyelids, otherwise known as a black eye, is of course a common problem especially on Saturday nights in a general casualty department. Usually the presence of a black eye is an indication that the afflicted was smart enough to close his eye in time to avoid injury to the globe. It is unusual to find damage to the eyes after Saturday night fistfights, unless a weapon was involved. Broken beer glasses produce devastating injuries to the eyes as well as to the eyelids.

Injuries to the Orbit

Blows on the side of the cheek and across one or other eye occur in industrial or road-traffic accidents. The most common type is the "blow out fracture". Here the globe and contents of the orbit are forced backward causing fracture of the orbital floor and displacement of bone downwards into the antrum. The inferior rectus muscle becomes tethered so that there is limitation of upward movement. The infraorbital nerve may also be injured producing anaesthesia of the skin of the cheek. Once the surrounding swelling has subsided, the posterior displacement of the globe becomes obvious and the globe of the eye itself often shows evidence of contusion. A considerable improvement from the functional and cosmetic point of view can be obtained by positioning a plastic implant in the floor of the orbit after freeing the prolapsed tissue.

Fractures of the skull, which extend into the orbit, may be accompanied by retro-orbital haemorrhage and proptosis. Cranial nerve palsies affecting the ocular movements are also commonly seen in this type of injury and the vision may be affected by optic nerve damage. A blow on the eye may result in sudden blindness with at first no other evidence of injury (apart from an afferent pupillary defect), but subsequently the optic disc becomes pale and atrophic after two or three weeks.

Radiational Injuries

The eyes may be exposed to a wide range of electromagnetic radiation from the shorter wavelength ultraviolet rays through the wavelengths of visible light to the longer infrared waves, X-rays and microwaves. X-rays pass straight through the eye without being focused by the optical media and, in large enough doses may cause generalised damage. It is important to realise that therapeutic but not diagnostic doses of X-rays tend to cause cataracts and the eye must be suitably screened during treatment. Excessive doses of X-rays also cause stenosis of the lacrimal canaliculi and retinal neovascularisation. As one might expect, visible light does not normally damage the eyes, although an intense light source may be absorbed by the pigment epithelium behind the retina and converted to heat, producing a macula burn. After eclipses of the sun there are usually a number of patients who arrive in the casualty departments of eye hospitals with macular oedema and sometimes serious permanent impairment of visual acuity. Sun gazing with consequent retinal damage has been reported after taking LSD. The laser beam provides a source of intense light, which is used widely in ophthalmology as a deliberate means of producing gentle burns in the retina or making holes in the lens capsule after cataract surgery. Ultraviolet rays, which are shorter than visible light, do not normally penetrate the eye but

in large enough doses produce burns of the eyelids and cornea. On the skin this is seen as erythema and later pigmentation, and on the cornea a punctate keratitis is seen with the slit-lamp. Ultraviolet damage of this kind is seen after gazing with unprotected eyes at welder's arcs, after exposure of the eyes to sunray lamps, and after exposure to the sun under certain conditions such as in snow on mountain tops. All these types of injury show a delayed effect, the symptoms appearing 2 or 3 h after exposure and lasting for about 48 h. There is usually severe pain and photophobia so that it may not be possible to open the eyes, hence the term "snow blindness". The use of locally applied steroid and antibiotic drops hastens recovery.

Unlike ultraviolet light, infrared rays penetrate the eye and can cause cataract. A specific kind of thermal cataract has been well described in glassblowers and furnace workers but this is now rarely seen due to the use of protective goggles. Microwaves, in the form of diathermy, can cause cataract but the eye must be in the path of the beam if damage is to occur, and microwave ovens would not be expected to be dangerous in this respect. Concern is quite often expressed in the press or elsewhere about the possibility of radiation damage to the eyes from visual display units (VDUs). Such damage has never been demonstrated any more than it has from the face of a television set. Someone not used to working with a VDU who is suddenly made to spend several hours a day in front of one may experience eyestrain especially if incorrect spectacles are worn.

Chemical Injuries

These are quite common but usually not severe enough to warrant hospital attention. In industrial premises there is now nearly always a first-aid post with facilities to wash out the eyes. Plain water or a salt solution is the best fluid to use and valuable time may be lost if washing is delayed in order to search for a specific antidote. More severe burns can result from the catalysts used in the manufacture of plastics or from alkalis such as caustic soda. One needs to be particularly wary of alkali burns, since they may not seem so severe at first until the full effect of the chemical reaction on the tissues has occurred. Acid burns as from exploding car batteries are quite commonly seen in large casualty departments but are usually less severe.

Section IV

Problems of the Medical Ophthalmologist

Testing Visual Acuity 17

Measuring Visual Acuity

Measurement of visual acuity is the most important test of vision performed by the doctor and yet it is surprising how often the non-specialist omits it in examination. It has already been shown that the differential diagnosis of the red eye can be simplified by noting the vision in the affected eye. After injuries of the eye it is just as important to note the vision in the uninjured eye as it is to note that in the injured eye. Simple measurement of visual acuity is of course, of limited value without a knowledge of the spectacle correction or whether the patient is wearing the appropriate spectacles. The best-corrected visual acuity therefore needs to be recorded for each eye. This corrected visual acuity can be estimated with a pinhole.

Measuring the visual acuity means measuring the function of the macula, which is of course only a small part of the whole retina. A patient may have grossly impaired visual acuity and yet have a normal visual field enabling him or her to walk about and lead a normal life apart from being able to read. This state of affairs is seen in patients with age-related macular degeneration and can be compared with the situation in which a patient has grossly constricted visual fields but normal macular function, as is sometimes seen in retinitis pigmentosa or advanced chronic simple glaucoma. Here the patient appears to be blind, being unable to find his or her way about, but he may surprise the ophthalmologist by reading the test type from top to bottom once found.

The simplest way to measure visual acuity might be to determine the ability to distinguish two points when placed very close together. Such a method was supposed to have been used by the Arabs when choosing their horsemen. They chose only those who were able to resolve the two stars which form the second "star" in the tail of the Great Bear constellation. A point source of light such as a star, although it is infinitely small, forms an image with a diameter of about 11 μm on the retina. This is because the optical media are not perfect and allow some scattering of the light. In practice, it is possible for a person with normal vision to distinguish two points apart if they are separated by 1 mm when placed 10 m away. Two such points would be separated by 2 μm on the retina. This might be surprising considering that a spot of light casts a minimum size of image of 11 μm due to scatter, but such an image is not uniform, being brighter in the centre than at the periphery. In fact, the resolving power of the eye is limited by the size of the cones, which have a diameter of 1.5 μm.

In the clinic the visual acuity is measured by asking the patient to read a standard set of letters, the Snellen chart. This is placed 6 m from the eye. The single large letter at the top of this chart is designed to be just discernible to a normally sighted person at a range of 60 m. If the patient's vision is so poor that only this and no smaller letter can be seen at 6 m, then the vision is recorded as the fraction "6/60". The normal-sighted person who can read the chart down to the smaller letters designed to be discerned at 6 m is recorded as having a visual acuity of 6/6. The normal range of vision extends between 6/4 and 6/9 depending on the patient's age.

The near visual acuity is also measured using a standard range of reading types and here care must be taken to ensure that the correct spectacles for near work are used if the patient is over the age of 45 years (Figure 17.1). Normally the results of testing the near visual acuity are in agreement with those for measuring distance vision providing the

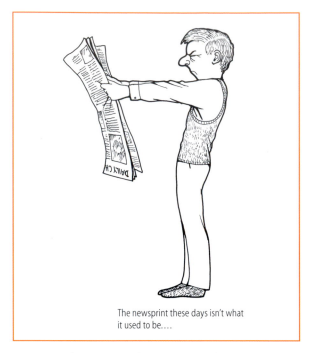

The newsprint these days isn't what it used to be....

Fig. 17.1.   Reading glasses in presbyopia.

correct spectacles are worn if needed. The visual acuity of each eye must always be measured by placing a card carefully over one eye and then transferring this to the other eye when the first eye has been tested. The visual acuity of both eyes together is usually the same or fractionally better than the vision of the better of the two eyes tested individually. In certain special circumstances the binocular vision may be worse than the vision of each eye tested separately.

A number of other tests have been developed to measure visual acuity in the non-literate patient. Infants below the reading age can be measured with surprising accuracy using the Stycar test. Here, letters of differing size are shown to the child, who is asked to point to the same letter on the card, which is given to him or her. Up to the age of 18 months or two years, the optokinetic drum may be used. This makes use of the phenomenon of optokinetic nystagmus produced by moving a set of vertically arranged stripes across the line of sight. When the stripes are sufficiently narrow, they are no longer visible and fail to produce any nystagmus. The eyes are examined using a graded series of stripes. This kind of test can be used to measure visual acuity in animals other than humans. The "E" test is a way of measuring the visual acuity of illiterate patients.

This is based on the Snellen type but the patient is presented with a series of letter "E"s of different sizes and orientations and is given a wooden letter "E" to hold in the hands. He is then instructed to turn the wooden letter to correspond with the letter indicated on the chart.

The Snellen type has the great advantage of being widely used and well standardised, but it must be realised that it is a measure of something more complex than simply the function of the macula area of the retina. It involves a degree of literacy and also speech, and testing shy children or elderly patients may sometimes be misleading.

One final way of measuring the visual acuity is by assessing the ability to resolve a grating. Here, the word "grating" refers to a row of black and white stripes where the black merges gradually into the white. Such a grating can be varied by altering either the contrast of black and white or the width of the stripes (the "frequency"). Thus for a given individual, the threshold for contrast and frequency (contrast sensitivity) can be measured. This type of test has certain theoretical advantages over standard methods but it is not widely used clinically as a routine.

Measuring for Spectacles

If a patient has not been recently tested for spectacles, then not only may the measurement of visual acuity be inaccurate, but the symptoms may be due to the need for a correct pair of glasses. The measurement, which determines the type of spectacles needed, requires skill developed by practice and the use of the right equipment. The most obvious way to measure someone for a pair of glasses is to try the effect of different lenses and ask the patient whether the letters are seen better with one lens or another. This is known as subjective testing and by itself it is not a very accurate method because some patients' observations as to the clarity of letters may be unreliable. Furthermore, a healthy young person may see quite clearly with a wide range of lenses simply be exercising the ciliary muscle. Fortunately the refractive error of the eye can be measured by an objective method and an answer can be reached without consulting the patient. The method entails observing the rate of movement of the shadow of the iris against the red reflex from the fundus of the eye after interposing different strengths of lenses (retinoscopy). In order to make an accurate measurement of the spectacle requirement, both objective and subjective refractions are performed and the results compared.

Objective Refraction

The patient is fitted with a spectacle trial frame into which different lenses can be slotted. In the case of young children it is usually advisable to instil a mydriatic and cycloplegic drop beforehand to eliminate focusing. The ophthalmologist then views the eye to be examined through an instrument known as a retinoscope, from a distance of about one arm's length. The red reflex can be seen and the instrument is then moved slightly so that the light projected from the retinoscope moves to and fro across the pupil. The shadow of the iris on the red reflex is then seen to move, and the direction and speed of movement depend on the refractive error of the patient. By interposing different lenses in the trial frame, the movement of the iris shadow can be "neutralised" and the exact refractive error determined. The trial frame can accommodate both spherical and cylindrical lenses so that the amount of astigmatism can be measured.

Subjective Refraction

Here, considerable skill is also needed because many patients become quite tense when being tested in this way and may not initially give accurate answers. Lenses both stronger and weaker than the expected requirement are placed in the trial frames and the patient is asked to read the letters of the Snellen chart and to say whether they are more or less clear. A number of supplementary tests are available which enable one to check the patients' answers. It can be seen that the word "refraction" refers to the total test for glasses, although the same word refers to the bending of the rays of light as they pass from one medium to another. Accurate refraction takes 10 or 15 min to perform, or longer in difficult cases and it is an essential preliminary to an examination of the eye itself.

Automated Refraction

In recent years attempts have been made to develop an automated system of refraction, and instruments are now commercially available. They are, however, still expensive and not always accurate when there are opacities in the optical media, or when the patient over-accommodates. One further way of assessing the refractive error without asking the patient any questions is by making use of the visually evoked response. This is the name given to the minute electrical changes detectable over the back of the scalp when the eyes are exposed to a repeated stimulus, usually a flashing chequer-board. When fine checks are viewed, interposing different lenses can modify the response. This method is of great interest but it is still not very reliable and takes time to perform.

Summary

Considering the importance of the measurement of visual acuity, it is not surprising that a number of tests have been developed for this, but the simple Snellen chart remains an essential part of any doctors' surgery. It must be remembered that this is a measure of function in the centre of the visual field only and it is possible to have advanced loss of peripheral vision with normal visual acuity as is seen sometimes in patients with chronic glaucoma or retinitis pigmentosa. The assessment of the rest of the visual field has also been standardised and a number of instruments have been developed to measure it. These have already been described in Chapter 3 together with various other measurements of different aspects of vision.

The Inflamed Eye 18

In an earlier chapter we have already seen that "the red eye" is an important sign in ophthalmology, and there are a number of reasons why the eye may become inflamed. When the exposed parts of the eye such as the conjunctiva and the cornea are the primary sites of inflammation, the cause is usually infection or trauma. Common examples are chronic conjunctivitis or a corneal foreign body. However, here we are going to consider a type of inflammation, which arises, deeper in the eye and primarily from the uvea. The uvea has a tendency to become inflamed for no apparent external reason and in this respect can be compared to a joint; indeed, there is a recognised association between uveitis and arthritis. In spite of the fact that the eye is open to microscopic examination, the exact cause of uveitis is usually obscure, although there is evidence to indicate a relationship with other kinds of autoimmune disease.

Uveitis can be divided into anterior or posterior uveitis; anterior uveitis is the same entity as iridocyclitis, and posterior uveitis is the same as choroiditis. Apart from the uvea, the sclera and the episclera (that is, the connective tissue deep to the conjunctiva and overlying the sclera) may also be affected by similar inflammatory changes.

Anterior Uveitis

Symptoms

The patient suffering from acute anterior uveitis is usually aware that there is something seriously amiss with the eye. The vision is blurred and the eye aches and may often be extremely painful. Photophobia is usual and often pain on focusing on near objects is a feature. The age incidence is wide but anterior uveitis is commonly seen in the third and fourth decades of life, and every eye casualty officer becomes very familiar with this particular form. When the disease presents for the first time in the elderly, the underlying cause is likely to be different and age provides an important diagnostic feature. Acute anterior uveitis usually appears quite suddenly over a period of about 24 h and then resolves on treatment in two or three weeks; however, it may last as long as six weeks. A further exacerbation may occur during this period and there is a strong tendency towards recurrence after a few months or several years in the same or the other eye.

Signs

The eye is red, but of particular importance is the presence of a pink flush around the cornea (the ciliary flush) which indicates an inflammatory process either in the cornea or within the anterior chamber of the eye itself. The pupil is small because the iris sphincter goes into spasm. Thus the pupil of iritis is small and treatment is aimed at making it larger, whereas the pupil of acute glaucoma is large and treatment is aimed at making it smaller. Unless there is secondary glaucoma, the cornea remains bright and clear, but with a pen torch it may be possible to see that the aqueous looks turbid. That is to say, a beam of light shone through the aqueous resembles a beam of sunlight shining through a dusty room (Figure 18.1). Normally, of course, the aqueous is crystal clear even when examined with the microscope.

The presence of an occasional cell in the aqueous may be normal, especially if the pupil has been

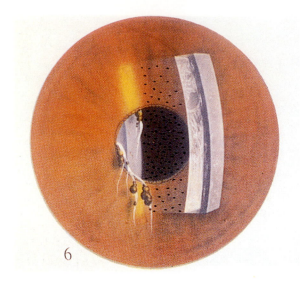

Fig. 18.1.   Flare.

dilated for some other reason, but suspicion should be raised if more than three or four cells are seen. In fact the early diagnosis of anterior uveitis can entail very careful slit-lamp examination. It is usual to discriminate between the presence of cells in the aqueous and the presence of flare. The latter reflects a high protein content and is a feature of more long-standing disease. Because there are convection currents in the aqueous, inflammatory cells are swept down the centre of the posterior surface of the cornea and become adherent to it, often forming a triangular-shaped spread of deposits known as keratic precipitates, or "KP"s (Figure 18.2). The microscopic appearance of the KP is determined by the type of cells. If a granulomatous type of inflammatory reaction is taking place involving epithelioid cells and macrophages, then the KP may be large, resembling oil droplets ("mutton fat KP"). This form of KP is seen in uveitis associated with sarcoidosis and also tuberculosis and leprosy. When the inflammation is non-granulomatous, a fine dusting of the posterior surface of the cornea may be evident. KPs tend to become absorbed but they may remain more permanently as pigmented spots on the endothelium.

Anterior uveitis is often associated with the formation of adhesions between the posterior surface of the iris and the lens. These are called posterior synechiae and become evident when attempts are made to dilate the pupil since parts of the iris remain stuck to the pupil giving it an irregular appearance. In severe cases of anterior uveitis, pus may collect in the anterior chamber to the extent that a fluid level may be seen where the layer of pus has formed inferiorly. This is known as hypopyon – literally, "pus below' (Figure 18.3). A hypopyon is an indication of severe disease in the eye and the patient should be treated in hospital. Hypopyon tends to occur in certain specific types of anterior uveitis. It is occasionally seen in elderly diabetics with inadequately treated corneal ulcers, particularly those with vascular occlusive disease. It is also seen in Behçet's disease, which is a rare disorder characterised by hypopyon uveitis, and ulceration of

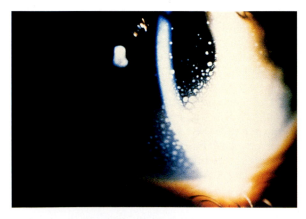

Fig. 18.2.   Keratic precipitates.

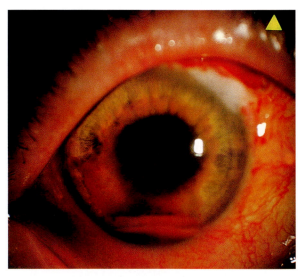

Fig. 18.3.   Hypopyon. In addition there are red blood cells and fibrinous exudate in the anterior chamber (with acknowledgement to Professor H. Dua).

the mouth and genitalia. A hypopyon is occasionally seen following cataract surgery and in such cases may be infective or non-infective in origin. It is fortunately a rare complication of modern cataract surgery and the use of intraocular acrylic lenses.

Complications

The visual prognosis of acute anterior uveitis as commonly seen in young people is usually good unless recurrences are frequent. Chronic uveitis is more prone to complications. Secondary glaucoma may cause serious problems and a careful check on the intraocular pressure must be maintained. The rise in intraocular pressure may be due to direct obstruction of the aqueous outflow by inflammatory cells or by the presence of adhesions between the peripheral part of the iris and the posterior surface of the cornea (peripheral anterior synechiae). Sometimes, especially when treatment has been inadequate, the posterior synechiae sticking the pupil margin to the anterior surface of the lens become extensive enough to obstruct the passage of aqueous through the pupil. The iris bulges forwards giving the appearance known as iris bombe. Secondary glaucoma may also result from the use of topical steroids in predisposed individuals.

Cataract is a further serious complication, which may appear after repeated attacks of anterior uveitis. It nearly always first affects the posterior subcapsular zone of the lens and unfortunately interferes with the vision at an early stage.

Causes

For the majority of patients who present to eye outpatient departments with this condition, no specific cause is found. However, there are many known causative agents. The ophthalmologist is obliged to exclude at least some of these even though he or she knows that more often than not a negative result will be obtained. It is necessary to explain this to patients otherwise considerable anxiety may be created by the fact that "no cause can be found" for their complaint. When we say no cause can be found we really mean that there is no evidence of any associated systemic disease and this should be of some reassurance to the patient.

It has already been mentioned that it can be helpful to consider the age of the patient when trying to eliminate the possibility of underlying systemic disease. Uveitis is very rare in young children,

but when seen, the possibility of juvenile rheumatoid arthritis must be borne in mind. In young adults sarcoidosis, gonorrhoea, Reiter's disease and ankylosing spondylitis are all recognised associations. In earlier years tuberculosis was very high on the list of suspected causes but this would appear to be a less common cause nowadays. Herpes simplex and zoster may also cause anterior uveitis. Septic foci in adjacent structures, such as dental sepsis or sinusitis, have also been under suspicion but these are now thought to be unimportant. In the case of the elderly, the onset of anterior uveitis may prove to be a recurrence of previous attacks and the same underlying causes must be suspected, but here there is also the possibility of lens-induced uveitis associated with by hypermature cataract. Three other types of anterior uveitis must be mentioned at this stage.

Sympathetic Ophthalmia

This is a rare, but dramatic, response of the uvea in both eyes to trauma. The significance of the condition rests in the fact that although the trauma has only affected one eye, the inflammatory reaction occurs in both. It may follow perforating injuries, especially when uveal tissue has become adherent to the wound edges. Occasionally it may occur following intraocular surgery. The injured eye, which is referred to as the "exciting eye", remains severely inflamed and, after an interval of between two weeks and several years, the uninjured eye ("sympathising eye") becomes affected. The inflammation in the sympathising eye usually starts in the region of the ciliary body and spreads anteriorly and posteriorly. It is granulomatous. Careful wound toilet and repair may probably prevent many cases, as can also removal of blind, painful and inflamed eyes within the critical two-week period following injury.

Heterochromic Iridocyclitis

This type of anterior uveitis presents in 20 to 40 year olds and is usually unilateral. The vision becomes blurred and the iris becomes depigmented. The eye usually remains white, the inflammatory reaction is low grade and chronic and posterior synechiae do not develop. The inflammation does not usually respond at all to treatment. Cataracts and chronic glaucoma occur very commonly. The condition has been mimicked by denervating the sympathetic supply of the eyes in experimental animals and it seems possible that there may be a neurological cause, unrelated and distinct from other types of uveitis.

Pars Planitis (Intermediate Uveitis)

This refers to a low-grade inflammatory response, which is seen in young adults. It affects both eyes in up to 80% of cases, although the severity may be asymmetrical. There is minimal evidence of anterior uveitis and the patient complains of floating spots in front of the vision. Inspection of the fundus reveals vitreous opacities and careful inspection of the peripheral retina shows whitish exudates in the overlying vitreous. A mild to moderate peripheral retinal phlebitis may occur. The condition runs a chronic course and occasionally may be complicated by cataract, cystoid macular oedema and tractional retinal detachment. The cause is unknown.

Treatment and Management

Once the diagnosis has been made, it is usual to embark on a number of investigations, guided in part by the history and taking into account especially any previous chest or joint disease. An X-ray of chest, and a blood count including measurement of the ESR are routine in most clinics, but the expense of further investigations is now often spared if the patient appears completely fit and well in other respects. The history and background of the patient may lead one to suspect the possibility of venereal disease. In the case of some infective types of anterior uveitis, the diagnosis is made before the uveitis appears because the condition occurs as a secondary event. This is the case following herpes simplex keratitis and also in patients with herpes zoster affecting the upper division of the Vth cranial nerve.

The treatment involves the administration of local steroids and mydriatic drops. When the condition is severe, a subconjunctival injection of steroid should be given and relief of symptoms may be further achieved by local heat in the form of a warm compress. Atropine is the mydriatic of first choice except in the mildest cases when homatropine or cyclopentolate drops may be used. Steroid drops should be administered every hour during the acute stage and then gradually tailed off over a period of a few weeks. Systemic steroids are not usually indicated and should be reserved for those cases in which the sight becomes seriously jeopardised. If any under-lying systemic disease is identified, then of course this should also be treated if effective treatment is available. The proper management of anterior uveitis demands the expertise of a specialist ophthalmologist and, when the condition is affecting both eyes, it may be preferable to admit the patient to hospital.

A special word of warning is needed for those patients who have undergone previous intraocular surgery. For these patients what is normally a mild infective conjunctivitis may lead to intraocular infection. The development of anterior uveitis, weeks, even years, after the operation, can indicate disastrous consequences if urgent and intensive antibiotic treatment is not applied.

Posterior Uveitis

Symptoms

When the choroid, as opposed to the ciliary body and iris, becomes inflamed, the eye is not usually painful or red and the patient complains of severe blurring or loss of vision. If the focus of choroiditis remains peripheral, then the disease may remain unnoticed, as is witnessed by the relatively frequent observation of isolated healed foci in the fundi of asymptomatic patients. Often the inflammation spreads from choroid to retina the then to the vitreous. When this happens the vision becomes markedly blurred, even when the original focus is remote from the macula region. Alternatively the inflammation may originate from the retina and spread to involve the choroid and vitreous subsequently. Choroiditis at the macula itself usually leads to permanent loss of central vision.

Signs

In its early stages, choroiditis may be seen as a grey or yellowish raised area which may be discrete or multiple and anywhere in the fundus. A cellular reaction may appear in the overlying vitreous, seen as localised misting with the ophthalmoscope, and eventually the whole vitreous may become clouded, obscuring any view of the fundus and the original site of inflammation.

The patient usually presents at this stage so that the origin of the problem only becomes apparent after the inflammation has subsided. Retinitis manifests as an indistinct white cloudy area. When a

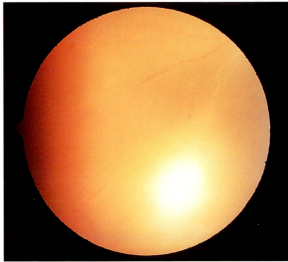

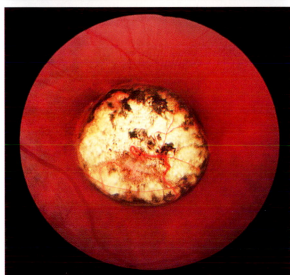

Fig. 18.4. Chorioretinitis: **a** active with hazy vitreous; **b** inactive scar.

nearly always occurs acutely over a period of hours, whereas the cloudiness following uveitis takes a few days to develop.

Examination of the vitreous with the slit-lamp can reveal whether the vitreous is filled with inflammatory cells or red cells. Retinal vasculitis may occur. A predominantly arteriolar inflammation may indicate a viral cause whereas venous involvement is more common with other aetiologies. Optic nerve inflammation or oedema may also occur.

Causes

As in the case of anterior uveitis, it is often impossible to pinpoint any systemic cause and the condition seems to be confined to the eye. However, a number of systemic associations have been recognised and often are related to specific types of posterior uveitis.

Toxoplasmosis

Toxoplasma gondii is a parasite, a protozoan carried by cats. Humans and other intermediate hosts may be infected. In the adult the acquired infection is usually mild. A severe form of acquired ocular toxoplasmosis has been recognised. In such cases there has been contact with wild cats in stables. In the case of infected pregnant mothers the child *in utero* may be infected by the more severe congenital form of the disease. The organism enters the brain as well as the eyes and may cause mental deficiency and epilepsy. A characteristic type of calcification is seen on skull X-ray or CT scan. In the eye a focal type of choroiditis often affects both eyes and this is usually at the posterior pole in the (macular region). Histologically the toxoplasma organism is found in the eye lesions. The diagnosis may be confirmed by sending some blood for serological tests. Four such tests are currently in use clinically: the toxoplasma dye test, indirect fluorescent antibody test, haemagglutination test and enzyme-linked immunosorbent assay (ELISA). These tests must be interpreted carefully because a high proportion of the population becomes infected at some point and the positive results increase with age, even in those with no clinical evidence of infection. For this reason the diagnosis may be less easy in acquired toxoplasmosis where evidence of systemic involvement may be slight or absent. It has been shown that there is a higher incidence of positive dye tests in patients with posterior uveitis than in the normal population, but in an individual case it is often necessary

patch of choroiditis heals, the margins become pigmented and a white patch of bare sclera remains. This is the result of atrophy of the pigment epithelium and choroid (Figure 18.4). Sometimes larger choroidal vessels survive as a clearly seen network overlying the white sclera surrounded by a pigment halo. During the active stage, inspection of the vitreous with the slit-lamp reveals the presence of cells and very often the anterior chamber also contains cells. Posterior uveitis comes into the differential diagnosis of a white eye with failing vision. When the vitreous becomes cloudy the condition must be distinguished from vitreous haemorrhage. The latter to demonstrate a changing titre in order to confirm the diagnosis. The most specific of these tests is the ELISA.

All the currently available antitotoxoplasma treatments have potentially serious side-effects. Therefore not all active toxoplasma retinochoroiditis lesions require treatment. Such treatment is required only if an active lesion involves or threatens the fovea and/or optic nerve. Treatment is also required when there is severe vitritis.

A combination of pyrimethamine and sulphadiazine has been recommended, but such treatment may cause a serious fall in the white cell count. An alternative antimicrobial treatment is clindamycin. This needs to be given with a sulphonamide in order to reduce the risk of colitis. It is generally accepted that systemic steroids have some beneficial effect and may help to clear the vitreous more rapidly, but this treatment should be given only with antimicrobial cover. Steroids on their own will produce exacerbation or progression of the chorioretinitis. In fact the majority of cases resolve spontaneously, leaving more or less chorioretinal scarring at the macular region. Recurrences are fairly common and the fresh choroidal inflammation tends to arise at the edge of a previous scar.

Toxocariasis

Toxocariasis is caused by *Toxocara cati* (from cats) or *T. canis* (from dogs). This nematode has been found in the enucleated eyes of young patients with a severe type of chorioretinitis. It is a unilateral disease found in children who are in close contact with puppies or eat dirt (through faecal contamination). The vitreous tends to be filled with a white mass of inflammatory cells so that the presence of a tumour may be suspected (e.g. retinoblastoma). Endophthlmitis tends to develop in these cases and the sight of one eye may be completely lost. During the acute stage the peripheral blood may show an eosinophilia. Treatment is unsatisfactory and includes a combination of antihelminthic agent taken by mouth (thiobendazole or diethylcarbamazine) and steroids.

Tuberculosis

In former years this was considered to be a common cause of posterior uveitis, clinicians having been impressed by the number of patients with a previous history of tuberculosis. The relationship seems less likely now that tuberculosis has been almost eliminated from the population. However, this diagnosis must not be forgotten especially in the immunosuppressed patient. Choroidal tubercles are a well-described entity: these raised yellowish granulomatous foci were used as a diagnostic feature of miliary tuberculosis and occasionally chronic pulmonary tuberculosis. They are only seen in extremely ill patients and the yellowish tubercles become pigmented as they heal. Treatment is as for systemic tuberculosis.

Sarcoidosis

The eye is very frequently involved in sarcoidosis. Involvement usually takes the form of an anterior or posterior uveitis. The choroiditis is more often peripheral and accompanied by inflammatory changes in the retinal veins. Sheathing of the veins may be seen and the vision may be impaired by macular oedema. The inflammatory changes may be similar to those seen in pars planitis. When the diagnosis is suspected, the conjunctiva and skin should be searched for possible nodules, which may be biopsied, and an X-ray of the chest may reveal enlargement of the hilar lymph nodes. The management of the ophthalmological problem may involve treatment with local and systemic steroids but the opinion of a physician specialising in sarcoidosis is essential and should be sought before embarking on treatment.

Presumed Ocular Histoplasmosis

Histoplasmosis is a fungal infection (causative agent – *Histoplasma capsulatum*). Infection with this organism occurs throughout the world but is more common in the Mississippi Valley in the USA and does not occur in the UK. A severe pneumonitis may occur but most cases are asymptomatic.

Presumed ocular histoplasmosis (POHS) is not seen in patients with active histoplasmosis. The evidence for infection in the originally described cases was necessarily circumstantial – hence the expression "presumed ocular histoplasmosis". The syndrome consists of a certain type of haemorrhagic macular lesion (choroidal neovascularisation) combined with discrete foci of peripheral choroiditis and peripapillary scars.

Syphilis

Syphilis is a chronic infection caused by *Treponema pallidum*. Iridocyclitis occurs in patients with secondary acquired syphilis. It is a bilateral disease in which the iris vessels are particularly engorged. Chorioretinitis may be either multifocal or diffuse and involves the mid-periphery and peripapillary area. In the healed phase, perivascular bone spicule pigmentation may be seen similar to that observed in retinitis pigmentosa.

In congenital syphilis other possible features occur such as deafness and corneal scarring from previous interstitial keratitis. The scattered pigmentation in the fundus may suggest an inherited retinal degeneration but a careful family history together with electrodiagnostic testing of the eyes usually enables one to distinguish the two conditions. It is also important to carry out serological testing. The *T. pallidum* immobilisation test (TPI) and the fluorescent treponemal antibody test (FTABS) are the most sensitive and specific.

Behçet's Disease

Behçet's disease is a multisystem disease associated with human leucoctye antigen (HLA)-B5. It was originally thought to occur only in the Mediterranean area and Japan where the disease is most common. The disease is characterised by an obliterative vasculitis. The clinical syndrome consists of oral and genital ulceration in combination with recurrent uveitis and skin lesions. The uveitis consists of recurrent bilateral non-granulomatous anterior and/or posterior uveitis. Central nervous system involvement occurs as a very serious form of the disease.

Other Causes

A wide variety of infective agents have been shown to cause posterior uveitis on rare occasions. The leprosy bacillus and the coxsackie group of viruses are two examples chosen from many. Sympathetic ophthalmia has already been mentioned as a specific form of uveitis following injury. An especially rare but intriguing form of uveitis is known as the Vogt–Koyanagi–Harada syndrome in which is seen the combination of vitiligo, poliosis, meningoencephalitis, uveitis and exudative retinal detachments.

The Role of Autoimmunity in Uveitis

Although it has been long recognised that bacterial and viral infection may account for some cases of uveitis, it has also been recognised that the majority of cases fail to show any evidence of this. Furthermore, in many instances the eye disease may be associated with known autoimmune disease elsewhere in the body. There are several different ways in which the uvea might be expected to become the focus of an antigen–antibody reaction. A foreign agent such as a virus might reside in the uvea and cause an antibody response, which coincidentally involves uveal tissue, or, on the other hand, a foreign agent might react with specific marker on the cell membrane to produce a new active antigen. It is now recognised that patients who inherit certain of the human leucocyte antigens (HLA) are more susceptible to particular types of uveitis, for example the uveitis seen in ankylosing spondylitis and Reiter's disease (HLA-B27). It has been suggested that HLA may act as the specific marker in these cases. A further way in which the uvea might become the centre of an immune response concerns the question of self-recognition. It now appears that there is a mechanism in the body, which normally prevents antibodies in the serum from acting against our own tissues. This active suppression is maintained by a population of thymus-derived lymphocytes (T lymphocytes) known as T-suppressor cells. There is evidence to suggest that sympathetic ophthalmitis might arise from inhibition of the T-suppressor cells after uveal antigens have been introduced into the bloodstream. Patients with juvenile rheumatoid arthritis occasionally develop uveitis, whereas rheumatoid disease in adults is more commonly associated with the dry eye syndrome and episcleritis.

Management

Increased interest in immunological diseases in recent years, which has accompanied advances in tissue grafting and cancer research, has led to attempts to treat uveitis with means other than steroids. Immunosuppressive agents, for eample, cyclosporin A, tacrolimus, azathioprine, cyclophosphamide, are now sometimes used to supplement or replace steroids in difficult cases. If posterior uveitis is not due to any recognisable infective cause, it is usual to start treatment with systemic steroids if the visual acuity becomes significantly impaired or if the lesion is close to the macula. Large doses of systemic steroids are best administered on an inpatient basis, especially if the sight is threatened. This has the added advantage of allowing a more detailed pretreatment examination and investigations, and often the opinion of a general physician or immunologist may be valuable at this stage. Secondary glaucoma may also need to be treated and immuno-suppressive agents may be administered to resistant cases. When posterior uveitis keeps recurring at the edge of previous healed foci, laser coagulation has been used in selected patients with toxoplasma retinochoroiditis. The rationale of this treatment is to destroy any remaining encysted organisms.

Endophthalmitis and Panophthalmitis

When inflammatory changes in the posterior uvea extend into the vitreous and there is an extensive involvement of the centre of the globe, the patient is said to have endophthalmitis. Further extension of the inflammation into the anterior segment of the eye and into the sclera leads to panophthalmitis. Endopthalmitis is one of the feared results of infection after injury or surgery but it may prove reversible with intensive antibiotic treatment. When endophthalmitis and panophthalmitis are not prop-erly and aggressively treated, the sight is usually lost permanently and the eye begins to shrink.

Episcleritis and Scleritis

Both these conditions form part of the differential diagnosis of the red eye. The episclera is the connective tissue underlying the conjunctiva and it may become selectively inflamed, either diffusely or in localised nodules. Close inspection of the eyes shows that the inflammation is deeper than the conjunctiva and there is a notable absence of any discharge. The eye is red and may be gritty but not painful. Episcleritis is seen from time to time in the casualty department and the patient may be otherwise perfectly fit and well. Such cases tend to recur and some develop signs of dermatological disease. The condition responds to local steroids, but systemic aspirin may also prove effective. Scleritis is less common and more closely linked with rheumatoid arthritis and other collagen diseases. The eye is red (diffuse or localised) and painful. In severe cases the sclera may become eroded with prolapse of uveal tissue.

The Ageing Eye 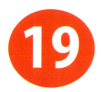 19

Although the eye and its supporting structures undergo a number of well-defined changes with age, the distinction between these involutional changes and disease is not always clear cut. For the elderly patient it is often reassuring to know that the problem is part of a "normal" process rather than the result of a specific illness and perhaps sometimes an artificial demarcation is drawn for the benefit of the patient.

The increase in number of elderly people presents problems in ophthalmology. A high proportion of elderly people instil drops into their eyes, either prescribed for them or as self-medication. It is important that adequate advice is received. Advising the elderly is often time consuming and may entail speaking to a younger relative or neighbour, but an adequate explanation of the disease or problems will avoid anxiety and probably the need for further subsequent unnecessary consultation.

The three commonest diseases of the elderly eye are cataract, glaucoma and age-related macular degeneration. The first can be cured, the second arrested or prevented, while the third generally tends to run a progressive course and treatment is unsatisfactory at present. Attempts to measure the incidence of these problems have produced a wide range of figures. Out of a population of elderly persons complaining of impaired vision about 30% turn out to have a cataract and a similar number to have age related macular degeneration, whereas 5% or less have chronic open angle glaucoma. Visual impairment due to glaucoma is more prevalent and occurs at an earlier age in blacks than in whites. Although there is an unexpectedly high incidence of cataract in patients with chronic simple glaucoma, the association of macular degeneration with cataract or glaucoma is more random.

Changes in the Eyes with Age

The External Eye

The eyelids tend to lose their elasticity and become less firmly opposed to the globe. The upper and lower lid margins become progressively lower so that whereas in the infant the upper lid may ride level with or slightly above the corneal margin, in an elderly subject the upper lid may cross a significant part of the upper cornea. An area of white may be seen between the lower margin of the cornea and the lower lid. Some limitation of the ocular movements is accepted as normal in the elderly, especially limitation of upward gaze. The conjunctiva tends to become more lax and a thin fold of conjunctiva may be trapped between the lids when blinking if this becomes excessive. In some elderly patients there is loss of connective tissue around the lacrimal puncta so that the opening is seen elevated slightly from the rest of the lid. Degenerative plaques are seen on the bulbar conjunctiva in the exposed region and the conjunctiva is especially prone to chronic inflammation.

The Globe

Arcus senilis is the name given to the circular white infiltrate seen around the margin of the cornea. The lens gradually loses it plasticity throughout life and this results in a progressive reduction in the focusing power of the eye. This loss of focusing ability is also contributed to by the progressive loss of ciliary muscle tone. A child may be able to observe details of an object held 5 cm from the eye, but as a result of hardening of the lens and weakening of ciliary muscle the nearest point at which an object can be kept in focus gradually recedes. This progressive degeneration tends to pass unnoticed until the eye is no longer able to focus to within the normal reading distance. This usually occurs at the age of 45 years if the eyes are otherwise normal, and the phenomenon is called presbyopia.

Some degree of opacity of the lens fibres is very common in old age and only when this becomes more extensive is the term "cataract" used. The pupil becomes smaller with age and does not show the wide range of adjustment to illumination seen in younger people.

The vitreous shows an increase in small opacities visible to the subject as "vitreous floaters". A more dramatic degenerative change, which occurs in a high proportion of normal individuals in the 60–70-year age group, is detachment of the vitreous. The formed part of the vitreous separates from the retina, usually above at first, leaving a fluid-filled gap between the retina and posterior vitreous face. Movement of the vitreous face may cause troublesome symptoms, for example flashing lights and floaters, but often a vitreous detachment goes unnoticed and is an incidental finding on examination of the eye. The important association between sudden vitreous detachment and subsequent retinal detachment has already been discussed in Chapter 13.

The appearance of the fundus also shows gradual changes; the retinal arterioles become straighter and narrower, as also do the venules. Colloid bodies or drusen are more commonly seen due to degenerative changes in Bruch's membrane and the pigment epithelium, and peripheral chorioretinal degeneration is more evident. The young retina is more shiny than the old retina and in the elderly the normal light reflex is less marked. The optic disc tends to become somewhat paler and a degree of optic atrophy is accepted by many clinicians as a senile change unrelated to disease.

Eye Disease in the Elderly

The prevalence of blindness increases with age. Prevalence and causes of blindness also varies from one community to another depending on the age structure of the population and environmental conditions. In England and Wales (1980), the prevalence of blindness was found to be 9/100,000 under five years of age and 2324/100,000 above 75 years.

A recent survey in the United States has shown that the incidence of cataract in the 45–64-year-old population is 5.6% for males and 2.1% for females. The incidence is slightly higher in the black population, and rises to 21.6% for males and 26.8% for females in the 65–75-year-old population. In the same age group (65–75 years) the incidence of age-related macular degeneration is 9.6% for males and 6.9% for females. Both these conditions are therefore very common and they demand time and medical expertise, both at the primary care level and in hospital.

With increasing longevity throughout the world especially in the developing countries, there will be a continuing increase in the number of blind people, especially those suffering from diseases related to age such as cataracts, glaucoma, and macular degeneration.

Age-related Macular Degeneration

Age related macular degeneration (AMD) is the commonest cause of incurable blindness in the elderly in western countries. It is a bilateral disease in which visual loss in the first eye usually occurs at about 65 years of age. The second eye is involved at the rate of 10% per annum.

Older patients with macular degeneration complain of blurring of their vision and inability to read. Younger or more observant patients notice that straight edges may look kinked. Usually one eye is considerably more affected than the other, although both eyes may be affected simultaneously. Because the degenerative process is limited to the macula, the peripheral field remains unaffected and the patient can walk around quite normally. Difficulty in recognising faces or in seeing bus numbers is also a common complaint. About a third of the patients give a family history of similar problems.

In the early stages of the condition, inspection of the fundus shows spots of pigment in the macular region. Drusen are also often seen (Figure 19.1). These are small round yellowish spots often scattered over the posterior pole. Unfortunately the word "drusen" has been used rather loosely in ophthalmology to refer to two or three types of swelling seen in the fundus. It is used to describe the very rare mulberry-like tumours seen around the optic nerve head in tuberose sclerosis and it is also used when referring to the multiple shiny excrescences seen on the optic disc as a congenital abnormality.

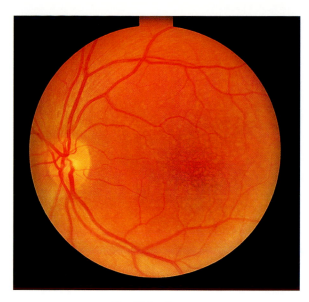

Fig. 19.1.   Drusen.

Drusen seen at the posterior pole of the eye as a senile change are also known as "colloid bodies" and perhaps this term is preferable. Under the microscope, colloid bodies are seen as a degenerative change in Bruch's membrane. Drusen may have varying degrees of hyperpigmentation. Most eyes with drusen maintain good vision, but a significant number will develop progressive atrophy of the retinal pigment epithelium (RPE) and choriocapillaris. This is inevitably associated with photoreceptor loss. [Figure 19.2] There is usually a moderate loss of vision. This atrophic change in the RPE, choroid and photoreceptors is referred to as "dry" AMD. This is because there is no leakage of fluid or bleeding into the retina or subretinal space.

In the "wet type" of macular degeneration a fan of new vessels arises from the choroid – choroidal neovascularisation (CNV). The growth of these new vessels seems to be important because they invade the breaks in Bruch's membrane. Serous or haemorrhagic exudate tends to occur and this may be either under the pigment epithelium or subretinal (Figure 19.3). A sudden loss of central vision may be experienced as the result of such an episode.

Management

No effective treatment is available for dry AMD. There is an increasing vogue for administering vitamins C and E, selenium, copper and zinc preparations to patients (orally). These substances are thought to reduce the damaging effects of light on the retina through their reducing and free-radical scavenging actions.

Some types/stages of wet AMD are treatable. However, the treatment for most eyes with wet AMD is unsatisfactory.

Controlled trials of the effect of laser photocoagulation of the choroidal new vessels have shown that this treatment is useful in extrafoveal CNV. Laser photocoagulation ablates the CNV. It is important that those cases that are likely to benefit from treatment are first identified. At the present time this entails photography of the fundus and fluorescein angiography, and infrared angiography with indocyanine green. Very often patients present at the stage when new vessels have already advanced across the macular region to the subfoveal area or where the fovea has already been permanently damaged by haemorrhage or exudate, making effective laser treatment impossible. Apart from photocoagulation, there are other treatment modalities, for example, radiotherapy, photodynamic therapy and drugs including thalidomide currently under investigation.

Practical measures can be taken in the management of these patients to alleviate their handicap. Telescopic lenses may be needed for reading or watching television and full consideration should be given to the question of blind registration. It is important to explain the nature of the condition and prognosis to the patient. This can alleviate considerable anxiety and fear of total blindness and help the patient come to terms with the problem. In most

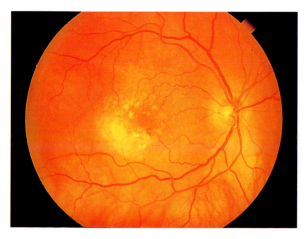

Fig. 19.2.   Dry macular degeneration.

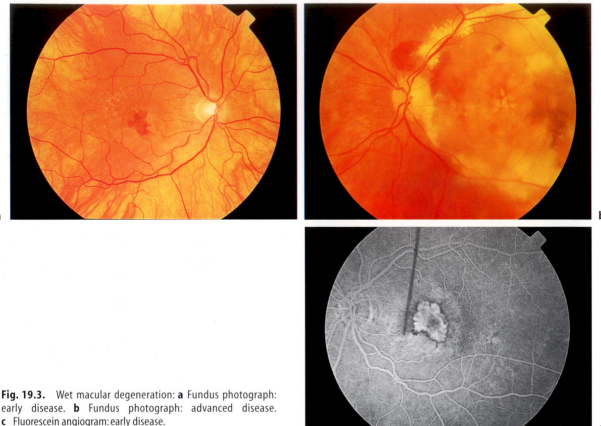

Fig. 19.3. Wet macular degeneration: **a** Fundus photograph: early disease. **b** Fundus photograph: advanced disease. **c** Fluorescein angiogram: early disease.

cases one eye is involved first, the other following suit after one to three years. The vision, as measured on the Snellen chart, progressively deteriorates to less than 6/60, but the peripheral field remains unaffected so the patient is able to find his or her way about, albeit with some difficulty.

Cataract

This common condition in the elderly eye has already been considered, but it is important that every physician can identify and assess the density of a cataract in relation to the patient's vision. The physician must realise the potential of cataract surgery in the restoration of vision. Cataract surgery is required only if vision is sufficiently reduced so far as to interfere with the patient's normal lifestyle. The contraindications for cataract surgery are few and even in extreme old age the patient may benefit. Surgery may be delayed if the patient has only one eye or if there is some other pathology in the eye, which is likely to effect the prognosis. The need for someone to assist the patient in

the instillation of eyedrops and the domestic chores during the post-operative period may require some attention but is not a contraindication. About one-third of the population aged over 70 years of age suffer from a cataract, but the quoted figures vary according to the diagnostic criteria. If an elderly person has an opaque lens, which obscures any view of the fundus with the ophthalmoscope, and the pupil reacts quickly, then he or she is likely to do well after surgery. It is useful to remember that the reading vision is usually fairly well preserved even when the cataract is quite dense, and if the patient is unable to read, there may be coincidental age-related macular degeneration, except if the cataract is of the posterior subcapsular type.

Glaucoma

The various types of glaucoma have also been considered already, and the reader would realise that glaucoma is simply the manifestation of a group of diseases each of which has a different prognosis and treatment. Chronic simple or open angle glaucoma is the important kind in the elderly because it often remains undiagnosed. The physician and optometrist can play an essential part in the screening of this disease by becoming familiar with the nature of glaucomatous cupping of the optic disc. About 1% of the population over the age of 55 years is thought to suffer from chronic simple glaucoma and the figure may rise to as high as 30% in those over 75 years. In most instances the treatment is very simple but requires the co-operation and understanding of the patient. The treatment is preventative of further visual loss rather than curative. Chronic simple glaucoma is best managed in an eye unit on a long-term basis. By this means the visual fields and intraocular pressure can be accurately monitored and the treatment adjusted as required.

Deformities of the Eyelids

Both entropion and ectropion are common in the elderly and a complaint of soreness and irritation in the eyes as well as watering should always prompt a careful inspection of the configuration of the eyelids. Entropion is revealed by pressing the finger down on the lower lid so that the inverted lid becomes everted again to reveal the lash line. Sometimes entropion may be intermittent and not present at the time of examination, but usually under these circumstances, there is a telltale slight inversion of the lid, which is made apparent by comparing the two sides. Ectropion is nearly always an obvious deformity due to the easy visibility of the reddened and everted conjunctiva, but slight degrees of ectropion are less obvious. The lower punctum alone may be slightly everted, causing a watering eye, and the symptoms may be relieved by applying retropunctal cautery to the conjunctiva.

Both ectropion and entropion respond very well to lid surgery and there is no reason why geriatric patients should put up with the continued discomfort and irritation when a complete cure is readily available. These lid deformities may recur sometimes and require further lid surgery, but careful surgery in the first instance should largely prevent this.

Temporal Arteritis

This condition, also known as giant cell arteritis, seen only in the elderly, may rapidly cause total blindness unless it is treated in time. The disease is more common than was originally supposed but it is

very rare under the age of 50 years. Medium-sized vessels, including the temporal arteries, become inflamed and the thickening of the vessel wall leads to occlusion of the lumen. Histologically the inflammatory changes are characterised by the presence of foreign body giant cells and the thickening of the vessel wall is at the expense of the inner layers so that the total breadth of the vessel may not be altered. In early disease, the inflammatory changes tend to be segmental so that a single biopsy of a small segment of the temporal artery does not always reveal the diagnosis.

Patients with temporal arteritis usually present in the eye department with blurring of vision or unilateral loss of vision. Typically these symptoms are accompanied by headache and tenderness of the scalp so that brushing the hair may be painful. Often there is low-grade fever and there may be aches and pains in the muscles and joints as well as other evidence of ischaemia in the brain and heart. Scalp ulceration and jaw claudication may occur. The blurring of vision is due to ischaemia of the optic nerve head or occasionally central retinal artery occlusion. The diagnosis rests largely on finding a raised ESR, elevated C-reactive protein (CRP) levels and a positive temporal artery biopsy in an elderly patient with these symptoms. Palpation of the temporal arteries reveals tenderness and sometimes thickening and the absence of pulsation is a useful sign. Polymyalgia rheumatica is a syndrome consisting of muscle pain and stiffness affecting mainly the proximal muscles without cranial symptoms.

Inspection of the fundus in a patient with visual symptoms shows pallor and often swelling of the optic nerve head and narrowing of the retinal

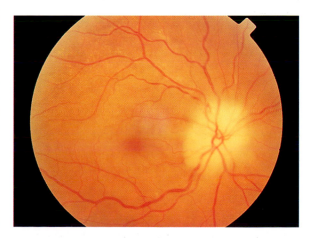

Fig. 19.4.   Giant cell arteritis: ischaemic optic neuropathy.

arterioles (Figure 19.4). Once the disease is suspected, a biopsy is essential and this should be done without delay. Treatment can be commenced immediately sometimes even before biopsy. However, it is advisable that the lag between starting treatment and biopsy is as short as possible (preferably less than two weeks). The symptoms disappear rapidly after administering systemic steroids, initially in a high dose (e.g. prednisolone 120 mg per day), and the dosage is then reduced rapidly according to the level of the ESR. Once the ESR is down to normal levels, a maintenance dose of systemic steroids is continued, if necessary for several months (18 months on average).

Temporal arteritis is recognised as a self-limiting condition. About one-quarter of all patients are liable to become blind unless adequate treatment is administered and in some instances extraocular muscle palsies causing diplopia and ptosis may confuse the diagnosis. For simplicity one might summarise the disease by saying it causes headache in patients aged over 70 years with an ESR over 70, who require treatment with over 70 mg of prednisolone.

Stroke

Patients who complain of visual symptoms after a stroke quite often have an associated homonymous hemianopia and the association between hemiplegia and homonymous hemianopia should always be borne in mind. A simple confrontation field test may be all that is required to confirm this in a patient with poor vision and normal fundi following a hemiplegic episode. The vertical line of demarcation between blind and seeing areas is very well defined and may cut through the point of fixation. Fortunately the central 2 or 3 degrees of the visual field are often spared. When there is the so called macular sparing, the visual acuity as measured by the Snellen chart may be normal. Patients tend to complain of difficulty in reading if the right homonymous field is affected rather than the left, and although they may be able to read individual words, they have great difficulty in following the line of print. Thus a patient with a right hemiplegia and a right homonymous hemianopia may have normal fundi and visual acuity of 6/6 and yet be unable to read the newspaper. The picture may be further complicated by true dyslexia and the patient may admit to being able to see the paper and yet be unable to make any sense of it. Dyslexia may be suspected if other higher functions such as speech have been affected by the stroke. One of the features of a homonymous hemianopic defect in the visual field is the patient's complete lack of insight into the problem, so that even a doctor may fail to notice it in himself. It is unusual for a homonymous hemianopia to show any signs of recovery, but once patients understand the nature of the handicap they may learn to adapt to it to a surprising degree.

The Child's Eye   20

How the Normal Features Differ from those in an Adult

At birth the eye is large, reaching adult size at about the age of two years. One might expect that before the eye reaches its adult size, it would be long sighted, being too small to allow parallel rays of light to be brought to a focus on the retina. In actual fact the immature lens is more globular and thus compensates for this by its greater converging power. None the less, more than three-quarters of children aged under four years of age are slightly hypermetropic. The slight change of refractive error which occurs as they grow compares with the more dramatic change in axial length from 18 mm at birth to 24 mm in the adult. The slight degree of hypermetropia seen in childhood tends to disappear in adolescence. Myopia is uncommon in infancy but tends to appear between the ages of six to nine years and gradually increases over subsequent years. The rate of increase of myopia is maximal during the growing years and this may often be a cause of parental concern.

The iris of the newborn infant has a slate-grey colour due to the absence of stromal pigmentation. The normal adult coloration does not develop fully until after the first year. The pupil reacts to light at birth but the reaction may be sluggish and it may not dilate very effectively in response to mydriatic drops. The fundus tends to look grey and the optic disc somewhat pale, deceiving the uninitiated into thinking that it is atrophic. The foveal light reflex, that is the spot of reflected light from the fovea, is absent or ill-defined until the infant is 4–6 months old. By six months the movement of the eyes should be well co-ordinated, and referral to an ophthalmol-ogist is needed if a squint is suspected. Once children learn to identify letters, at the age of four or five years, the Snellen chart can be employed to measure visual acuity, which by this age is normally 6/9 or 6/6. The Stycar test can be used for 3–4 year olds or sometimes younger children and a similar level of visual acuity is seen as soon as the child is able to co-operate with the test conditions. Stycar results tend to be slightly better than Snellen results when measured in the same child, perhaps because the Stycar test involves seeing a single letter rather than a line.

How to Examine a Child's Eye

The general examination of the eye has been considered already, but in the case of the child, certain aspects require special consideration. Before the age of three or four years, it may not be possible to obtain an accurate measure of the visual acuity, but certain other methods which attempt to measure fixation are available. The rolling ball test measures the ability of the child to follow the movement of a series of white balls graded into different sizes. Another test makes use of optokinetic nystagmus, which can be induced, by making the child face moving vertical stripes on a rotating drum. The size of the stripes is then reduced until no movement of the eyes is observed.

In practice, a careful examination of the child's ability to fix a light, and especially the speed of fixation, is helpful. The behaviour of the child may also be a helpful guide, such as, for example, the response to a smile or the recognition of a face. Sometimes grossly impaired vision in infancy is overlooked or interpreted as a psychiatric problem, but such an error an error can usually be avoided by careful ophthalmological examination. The reaction of the pupils is an essential part of any visual assessment. One of the difficulties in examining children is that they are rarely still for more than a few seconds at a time, and any attempts at restraint usually make matters worse. Before starting the examination it is useful to gain the child's confidence by talking about things that might interest him or her, not directly but in conversation with the parent. In fact, it is sometimes better to ignore the very anxious child deliberately during the first few minutes of the interview. Once the young patient has summed you up, hopefully in a favourable light, then a gentle approach in a quiet room is essential for best cooperation. The cover test can only be performed well under such conditions and once this has been done the pupils and anterior part of the eye can be examined, first with a hand lens but if possible with the slit-lamp microscope.

Fundus examination and measurement of any refractive error demand dilatation of the pupils and paralysis of accommodation. Cyclopentolate 1% or tropicamide 1% are both used in drop form for this purpose. The indirect ophthalmoscope is a useful tool when examining the neonatal fundus, the wide field of view being an advantage in these circumstances. If the infant is asleep in the mother's arms, this may be beneficial because it is a simple matter to raise one eyelid and peer in without waking the patient. In the case of children between the ages of three and six years, fundus examination can be more easily achieved by sitting down and asking the standing patient to look at some spot or crack on the wall while the optic disc is located. On some occasions the child has become too excited or anxious to allow a proper examination and here one may have to decide whether it is reasonable to postpone the examination for a week or whether the matter seems urgent enough to warrant proceeding with an examination under anaesthesia.

A casualty situation, which occurs from time to time, is when a child is brought in distress with a suspected corneal foreign body or perhaps a perforating injury. Here it is simplest to wrap the patient in a blanket so as to restrain both arms and legs and then examine the cornea by retracting the lids with retractors. Particular care must be taken when examining an eye with a suspected perforating injury in view of the risk of causing prolapse of the contents of the globe. Any ophthalmological examination demands placing one's head close to that of the patient and this can alarm a child unless it is done sufficiently slowly and with tact. It is sometimes helpful to make the child listen to a small noise made with the tongue or ophthalmoscope to ensure at least temporary stillness.

Screening of Children's Eyes

In an ideal world all children's eyes would be examined at birth by a specialist and again at six months to exclude congenital abnormalities and amblyopia. This is rarely achieved, although most children in the UK are examined by a non-specialist at these points. Most children are also screened routinely in school at the age of six years, and any with suspected poor vision are referred for more detailed examination. A further examination is often conducted at the age of nine or 10 years and again in the early teens. The commonest defect to be found is refractive error, that is simply a need for glasses without any other problem. The ophthalmological screening is usually performed by a health visitor in the preschool years and a school nurse for older children.

Screening tends to include measurement of visual acuity alone but checking any available family history of eye problems would be very helpful. When there is a difference in the visual acuity of each eye, the screener should suspect the possibility of a treatable medical condition rather than just a refractive error.

A test of colour vision should also be included in the screening programme for older children and this can be conveniently done using the Ishihara plates. It is worth remembering that colour blindness affects 8% of men and 0.4% of women and it may have important implications on the choice of a job. It is also equally important to realise that colour blindness may vary considerably in degree and may often be so mild as to cause only minimal inconvenience to the sufferer.

Congenital Eye Defects

Lacrimal Obstruction

The watering of one or both eyes soon after birth is a common problem. The obstruction is normally at the lower end of the nasolacrimal duct where a congenital plug of tissue remains. Infection causing purulent discharge can be treated effectively by the use of antibiotic drops. Although the unpleasant discharge clears the eye continues to water as long as the tear duct is blocked. The mother can be shown how to massage the tear sac. This manoeuvre causes mucopurulent material to be expressed from the lower punctum when there is a blockage and can be used as a diagnostic test. If carried out regularly, this helps to relieve the obstruction. In most cases spontaneous relief of the obstruction occurs, but if this does not occur after about six to nine months, probing and syringing of the lacrimal passageway under general anaesthesia is an effective procedure, which can be done as a day case.

It is important to remember that a watering eye may be due to excessive production of tears as well as inadequate drainage, and in a child, a corneal foreign body or even congenital glaucoma may be mistaken for lacrimal obstruction by the unwary.

Epicanthus

This relatively minor defect at the medial canthus is formed by a bridge of skin running vertically. This is seen normally in some oriental races. In Europeans it usually disappears as the bridge of the nose develops, but its importance lies in the fact that it may give the misleading impression that a squint is present. Severe epicanthus can be repaired by a plastic procedure on the eyelids.

Ptosis

Congenital ptosis may be unilateral or bilateral and sometimes shows a dominant inheritance pattern. The ptosis may be associated with other lid deformities. Referral for surgery is indicated if there is significant head tilt and especially if the lid covers the visual axis. See Chapter 4 for more information about eyelid deformities.

Structural Abnormalities of the Globe

There are many different developmental abnormalities of the globe, but fortunately most of these are rare. Coloboma refers to a failure of fusion of the foetal cleft of the optic cup in the embryo. Coloboma of the iris is seen as a keyhole-shaped pupil and the defect may extend into the choroid, so that the vision may be impaired. Inspection of the fundus reveals an oval white area extending inferiorly from the optic disc.

Children may be born without an eye (anophthalmos) or with an abnormally small eye (microphthalmos). It is always important to find out the full extent of this type of abnormality and if the mother has noticed something amiss in the child's eye, then referral to a paediatric ophthalmologist is required without delay. Often a careful discussion of the prognosis with both parents is needed.

Aniridia (congenital absence of the iris) may be inherited as a dominant trait and can be associated with congenital glaucoma. The lens may be subluxated or dislocated from birth. This may be suspected if the iris is seen to be tremulous. This strange wobbling movement of the iris used to be seen in the old days after cataract surgery without an implant, but it is now still seen after injuries to the eye and signifies serious damage.

Congenital subluxation of the lens is seen as part of Marfan's syndrome (congenital heart disease, tall stature, long fingers, high arched palate). Congenital glaucoma has already been discussed in the chapter on glaucoma; it may be inherited in a dominant manner and is the result of persistent embryonic tissue in the angle of the anterior chamber. When the intraocular pressure is raised in early infancy, the eye becomes enlarged producing buphthalmos ("bull's eye"). This enlargement with raised pressure does not occur in adults.

Congenital Cataract

The lens may be partially or completely opaque at birth. Congenital cataract is often inherited and may be seen appearing in a dominant manner together with a number of other congenital abnormalities elsewhere in the body. The condition may also be acquired *in utero*, the best known example of this being the cataract due to rubella infection during the first trimester of pregnancy: remember the triad of congenital heart disease, cataract and deafness in this respect.

Minor degrees of congenital cataract are sometimes seen as an incidental finding in an otherwise normal and symptomless eye. The nature of the cataract usually helps with the diagnosis. The lens fibres are laid down from the outside of the lens throughout life. If the opaque lens fibres are laid down *in utero* then this opaque region can remain in the centre of the lens. Only when the cataract is very thick does it present as a white appearance in the pupil and often it is difficult to detect it. It is important to examine the red reflex and see whether the darker opaque lens fibres show up. The surgeon has to decide whether the vision of the child has been significantly affected and unless the cataracts are very dense it may be better to wait until the school years approach in order to obtain a more accurate measure of the vision.

Sometimes vision may turn out to be surprisingly good with apparently dense cataracts. The surgical technique is similar to that for cataract surgery in the adult. Before the introduction of lens implants the risk of developing a retinal detachment in later life was very high in these patients. When the cataract is unilateral, this presents a special case because the affected eye tends to be amblyopic thus preventing a useful surgical result.

Congenital Nystagmus

Children with congenital nystagmus are usually brought to the department because their parents have noticed that their eyes seem to be continuously wobbling about. Such abnormal and persistent eye movements may simply occur because the child cannot see (sensory nystagmus) or they may be due to an abnormality of the normal control of eye movements (motor nystagmus). It is important to distinguish congenital nystagmus from acquired nystagmus due to a space-occupying intracranial lesion.

Sensory Congenital Nystagmus

The roving eye movements are described as pendular, the eyes tending to swing from side to side. Examination of the eyes reveals one of the various underlying causes: congenital cataract, albinism, aniridia, optic atrophy, or other causes of visual impairment in both eyes. A special kind of retinal degeneration known as Leber's amaurosis may present as congenital nystagmus. The condition resembles retinitis pigmentosa, being a progressive degeneration of the rods and cones, and occurs at a very young age. It tends to lead to near blindness at school age.

Patients with congenital nystagmus usually need to be examined under general anaesthesia, and electroretinography (a technique that can detect retinal degenerations at an early stage) should be performed at the same time.

Motor Congenital Nystagmus

The exact cause of this type of nystagmus is usually never ascertained but a proportion of such cases show recessive inheritance. Other abnormalities may be present, such as mental deficiency, but many children are otherwise entirely normal. The nystagmus tends to be jerky, with the fast phase in the direction of gaze to the right or left. The distance vision is usually impaired to the extent that the patient may never be able to read a car number plate at 23 m. The near vision, on the other hand, is usually good enabling many patients with this problem to graduate through university.

Spasmus Nutans

This term refers to a type of pendular nystagmus, which is present shortly after birth and resolves spontaneously after one or two years. Like other forms of congenital nystagmus, it may be associated with head nodding.

Albinism

The lack of pigmentation may be limited to the eye, ocular albinism, or it may be generalised. The typical albino has pale pink skin and white hair, eyebrows and eyelashes. There is often congenital nystagmus. The optic fundus appears pale and the choroidal vasculature is easily seen. The iris has a grey–blue colour but the red reflex can be seen through it giving the iris a red glow. Albinism is inherited in a recessive manner and may be partial or complete. Albinos need strong glasses to correct their refractive error, which is usually myopic astigmatism. Dark glasses are also usually required because of photophobia. Tinted contact lenses may sometimes be helpful.

Other Diseases in Childhood

Abnormalities of Refraction

Nowadays children whose vision is impaired because they need a pair of glasses are usually discovered by routine school testing of their visual acuity. They may also present to the doctor because the parents have noticed them screwing up their eyes or blinking excessively when doing their homework. Some children can tolerate quite high degrees of hypermetropia without losing visual acuity simply by exercising their accommodation, and unless there appears to be a risk of amblyopia or squint, glasses may not be needed. By contrast, even slight degrees of myopia, if both eyes are affected, can interfere with school work. Myopia does not usually appear until between the ages of five and 14 years, and most commonly at about the age of 11 years.

Squint

This exceedingly common inherited problem of childhood has already been considered, but it is worth summarising some of the main features. All cases of squint require full ophthalmological examination because the condition may be caused by treatable eye disease, most commonly amblyopia of disuse. There is no reason why any patient, child or adult, should suffer the indignity of looking "squint eyed" because the eyes can be straightened by surgery. In spite of this, it is not always possible to restore the full simultaneous use of the two eyes (binocular vision). In general, the earlier in life that treatment is started, the better the prognosis.

Amblyopia of Disuse

This has been defined as a unilateral impairment of visual acuity in the absence of any other demonstrable pathology in the eye or visual pathway. This rather negative definition fails to explain that there is a defect in nerve conduction due to inadequate usage of the eye in early childhood.

The word "amblyopia" means blindness and tends to be used rather loosely by ophthalmologists. It is most commonly used to refer to amblyopia of disuse ("lazy eye") but it is also used to refer to loss of sight due to drugs. Amblyopia of disuse is very common and some patients even seem unaware that they have any problem until they suffer damage to their sound eye. This weakness of one eye results when the image on the retina is out of focus or out of position for more than a few days or months in early childhood or, more specifically, below the age of eight years. Amblyopia of disuse therefore arises as the result of a squint or a one sided anomaly of refraction, or it may occur as the result of opacities in the optical media of the eye. A corneal ulcer in the centre of the cornea of a young child may rapidly lead to amblyopia.

Once a clear image has been produced on the retina, either by the wearing of spectacles or other treatment, the vision in the weak eye may be greatly improved by occluding the sound eye. The younger the patient, the better are the chances of improving the vision by occlusion. Beyond the age of eight years it is unlikely that any significant improvement can be achieved by this treatment and, by the same token, it is unlikely that amblyopia will appear after

the age of eight. An adult could suffer total occlusion of one eye for several months without experiencing any visual loss in the occluded eye.

Leucocoria

This term means "white pupil" and it is an important sign in childhood. There are a number of conditions that may produce this effect in early childhood. The important thing to realise is that if a mother notices "something white" in the pupil, the matter must never be overlooked and requires immediate investigation. The differential diagnosis includes congenital cataract, opaque nerve fibres in the retina, retinopathy of prematurity, endophthalmitis, some rare congenital abnormalities of the retina and vitreous and, not common but most important, retinoblastoma.

Retinopathy of Prematurity

In the early 1940s, premature infants with breathing difficulties began to be treated with oxygen, and 12 years elapsed before it was realised that the retinopathy seen in premature children was due to this very treatment. During the course of oxygen therapy in a premature infant, the retinal vessels become narrowed and the optic disc becomes pale. When the oxygen treatment is stopped, the retinal vessels become engorged and new vessels grow from the peripheral arcades in the extreme periphery of the fundus. This growth of abnormal vessels leads to vitreous haemorrhage, retinal detachment and fibrosis of the retina. The infant may rapidly become blind, although some are minimally affected.

The management of the condition now involves screening of those children at risk and monitoring of blood oxygen levels. When the condition occurs, treatment with cryotherapy to the peripheral retina has been shown to be beneficial. Now that children are being born at an earlier and earlier stage, it seems that extreme prematurity runs the risk of blindness from this cause even in the absence of supplementary oxygen.

Ophthalmia Neonatorum

It is important to realise that in the early part of this century, a large proportion of the inmates of blind institutions had suffered from ophthalmia neonatorum. The disease affects primarily the conjunctiva and cornea and is the result of infection by organisms resident in the maternal birth passage. The gonococcus was the most serious cause of blindness but a number of other bacteria have been incriminated including staphylococci, streptococci and pneumococci. It has also been shown that chlamydial infection of the genital tract may lead to the same problem as may also infection by the herpes simplex virus. The blindness, which resulted from this condition, was so serious that any excessive discharge from the eyes has been a notifiable disease in this country since 1914.

Ophthalmia neonatorum is caused by unhygienic conditions at birth and its relative rarity nowadays is due to the fact that midwives are trained to screen for the condition. Bacterial conjunctivitis usually occurs between the second and fifth day after birth whereas chlamydial infection tends to occur a little later, between the sixth and tenth day. Purulent or mucopurulent discharge is evident and the eyelids may become tense and swollen so that it is difficult to open them and carry out the all important examination of the cornea. When the disease is suspected, the infant should be admitted to hospital and treated with penicillin drops every hour. Diagnosis is achieved by taking a conjunctival culture before treatment is started and by looking for the inclusion bodies of the chlamydial virus in a smear. The history of infection in the parents needs to be explored and managed by a genitourinary specialist.

Uveitis

Uveitis is are in childhood; it may take the form of choroiditis, sometimes shown to be due to toxoplasmosis or toxocara, or the form of anterior uveitis sometimes associated with Still's disease. The management of these cases is similar to that of the adult, but recurrences may result in severe visual loss in spite of treatment.

Optic Atrophy

One must be rather wary about the diagnosis of optic atrophy in very young children because the optic discs tend to look rather pale in normal individuals. Occasionally unilateral visual loss with or without a squint is found to be associated with pallor of the disc on one side. Confirmed optic atrophy, either unilateral or bilateral, requires a full neurological investigation. The causes of optic atrophy in childhood are numerous but the important ones may be listed as follows:

- optic atrophy without systemic disease
  - hereditary optic atrophy
  - drug toxicity
- optic atrophy with systemic disease
  - glioma of chiasm and craniopharyngioma
  - post-meningitic
  - post-traumatic after head injury
  - hydrocephalus
  - cerebral palsy
  - disorders of lipid metabolism.

Juvenile Macular Degeneration

This is a rare cause of progressive visual loss in children, the diagnosis being made perhaps once in a lifetime at primary care level. For this reason the diagnosis can easily be missed especially as the patient finds difficulty in reading but no difficulty in walking around. Some cases show dominant inheritance and so the family history can be important.

The Phakomatoses

The three conditions von Recklinghausen's neurofibromatosis, tuberose sclerosis (Bournville's disease) and von Hippel–Lindau disease are classed together under this name. They all involve the eye but may not become evident until later life. Often examination of the eye reveals the diagnosis. In von Recklinghausen's neurofibromatosis, multiple neurofibromata are seen on the skin and the eyelids may be enlarged and distorted. Gliomata may develop in the optic nerves and scattered pigment "café au lait" patches are seen in the skin. Brown nodules can be seen on the iris. In tuberose sclerosis, mental deficiency and epilepsy are associated with a raised nodular rash on the cheeks and mulberry like tumours in the optic fundus. Von Hippel–Lindau disease presents to the ophthalmologist as angiomatosis retinae. Vascular tumours appear in the peripheral retina, which may leak and expand and lead to detachment of the retina. Similar tumours may be present intracranially.

Systemic Disease and the Eye 21

Diabetes

Diabetes mellitus affects 1–2% of the UK population and the condition is more prevalent in other countries. Diabetic retinopathy is the commonest cause of legal blindness in patients between the age of 20 and 65 years such that about 1000 people are registered blind from diabetes per year in the UK. The management of diabetic eye disease has improved greatly over the past 20 years so that much of the blindness can now be prevented. In spite of this, most general practitioners are aware of tragic cases of rapidly progressive blindness in young diabetics. The more serious manifestations of diabetes in the eye tend to affect patients in the prime of life. The tragedy is even greater when one considers that this blindness is largely avoidable.

Diabetes is therefore the most important systemic (non-infective) disease which gives rise to blindness. Many diabetics remain free of eye problems, but a diabetic is 25 times more likely to become blind than any other member of the population.

When taking an eye history from diabetic patients, it is especially important to note the duration of the diabetes and the age of onset since the incidence of diabetic retinopathy is most related to the duration of diabetes. Other risk factors are listed in Table 21.1.

Table 21.1. Risk factors for diabetic retinopathy

- Age
- Duration of diabetes
- Smoking
- Hypertension
- Poor diabetic control
- Hyperlipidaemia
- Renal impairment
- Pregnancy

Diabetic retinopathy is extremely rare under the age of 10 years; it does not usually appear until the disease has been present for some years. Juvenile onset diabetics usually take longer to show eye changes than those with a late onset.

Although diabetic retinopathy is the most serious ocular complication, the eye may be affected in a number of other ways and it is convenient to consider the various ocular manifestations of diabetes in an anatomical manner beginning anteriorly.

Eyelids

It is usual to check the urine of patients presenting with recurrent styes but in practice it is unusual for diabetes to be diagnosed in this way. Xanthelasma of the eyelids is said to be slightly more common in diabetics.

Ocular Movements

Elderly diabetic patients are more prone to develop transient IIIrd and VIth cranial nerve palsies than non-diabetics of the same age group. Sometimes isolated IIIrd nerve palsy may be painful and the pupil is spared. A fasting blood sugar may be required in patients presenting with isolated IIIrd nerve palsies. Hypertension and arteriosclerosis need exclusion.

Cornea and Conjunctiva

Some diabetics have microcirculatory changes, for example, conjunctival vascular irregularity and dilatation. Corneal ulcers in diabetics may prove particularly troublesome. Minor trauma to the cornea may lead to the formation of indolent chronically non-healing or infected ulcers, which respond very slowly to intensive treatment with local anti-biotics. Inadequate treatment may lead to endophthalmitis and loss of the eye. This problem occurs especially in diabetics with severe vascular disease and typically in a patient who has had to have a gangrenous leg removed.

Anterior Chamber

A particular kind of iritis is occasionally seen in diabetics after cataract surgery when there is a severe plastic reaction. It is important that such cases are treated adequately to prevent the development of posterior synechiae, which will make subsequent fundal examination difficult. It is advisable therefore to use mydriatic drops (cyclopentolate) after cataract surgery in diabetics.

Iris

The iris itself often shows degenerative changes in chronic diabetics. The pupil may react sluggishly and fail to dilate very widely after the instillation of mydriatic drops. The surgeon can appreciate that pigment is easily lost from the iris when it is handled, and it is interesting that a characteristic vacuolation of the pigment epithelium lining the posterior surface of the iris is seen in histological sections. When diabetes seriously interferes with the circulation of the eye, the iris may become covered on its anterior surface by a fibrovascular membrane. To the naked eye, the iris takes on a pinkish colour, but examination with the slit-lamp microscope or a magnifying lens soon reveals the minute irregular blood vessels on its surface. The appearance is

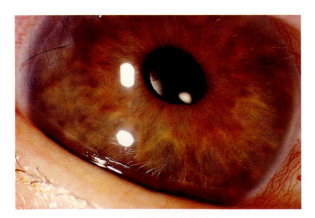

Fig. 21.1   Rubeosis iridis.

known as "rubeosis iridis" or neovasclarisation of the iris (Figure 21.1). Neovascular glaucoma occurs once the rubeosis involves the anterior chamber angle. If left untreated very few eyes with rubeosis iridis retain useful sight. The iris should be examined carefully before pupillary dilation.

Lens

It was mentioned in an earlier chapter that diabetics tend to develop senile cataracts at an earlier stage than normal. Cataracts once developed also progress more quickly in diabetics compared to non-diabetics. In addition, a rapidly advancing type of cataract is seen in young poorly controlled patients. This is a true diabetic cataract. This cataract is bilateral and consists of snowflake posterior or anterior opacities, matures rapidly and is similar to the rare cataract seen in starvation from whatever cause. The routine testing of urine of patients with cataracts produces a good return of positive results, making this an essential screening test.

It was also mentioned that the refractive power of the lens might change in response to a rise in the blood sugar level. This results from increased hydration of the lens in patients with high uncontrolled blood sugar levels. Undiscovered diabetics quite often become short-sighted due to this so-called index myopia. They may then obtain some distance glasses and subsequently consult their doctor, who treats their diabetes. By this time the glasses are made and, of course, turn out to be unsatisfactory, because the index myopia may improve with treatment. In some instances index myopia proves irreversible, being the first sign of cataract formation.

Retina and Vitreous

Diabetic retinopathy is the most serious complication of diabetes in the eye and often reflects severe vascular disease elsewhere in the body. There are two kinds of diabetic retinopathy: background and proliferative. Background retinopathy is very common when diabetes has been present for some years and is less of a threat to the sight than the proliferative variety. Diabetic maculopathy is a special form of retinopathy that may occur with either background or proliferative disease. It is important that the doctor is able to recognise diabetic retinopathy and especially important that he or she should be familiar with the warning signs that indicate proliferative changes and significant maculopathy.

Diabetic retinopathy is essentially a small vessel disease affecting the retinal precapillary arterioles, capillaries and venules. The larger vessels may be involved. The vascular disease may take the form of vascular leakage or closure, with resultant ischaemia, or both.

Background Retinopathy

There are usually no ophthalmic symptoms initially, but inspection of the fundi of most diabetics who have had the disease for ten years or more reveals, at first, a few microaneurysms. They are often on the temporal side of the macula but often scattered over the posterior pole of the fundus (Figure 21.2). These may come and go over months and the overall picture may be unchanged for several years. The vision is not affected unless the microaneurysms are clustered round the macular region and leak fluid resulting in macular oedema. Exudates are also seen and these tend to form rings around areas of diseased vessels, although only one part of the ring may be present at any given point. These are yellowish white deposits with well-defined edges, which are the result of precipitation of leaked lipoproteins from diseased blood vessels.

Capillary dilatation is a more subtle sign of diabetic retinopathy. Haemorrhages, which may be small ("dot") or large blot, result from the venous end of capillaries and are in the deep retina. Flame-shaped haemorrhages may also occur in the nerve fibre layer. "Cotton-wool" spots represent axoplasmic accumulation adjacent to microinfarction of the retinal nerve fibre layer. They are greyish white with poorly defined fluffy edges. Histological examination of diseased retina has shown areas of capillary closure and capillary microaneurysms. The vessel walls have thickened basement membranes and loss of mural cells (pericytes) (Figure 21.3).

Proliferative retinopathy is typically seen in poorly controlled diabetics (usually type I diabetes). The situation may become very bad very quickly and it is important to be able to recognise the warning signs, which occur before proliferation. There are three of them: a large number of dark blot haemorrhages, irregular calibre and dilatation of the retinal veins (beading) and finally, the presence of intraretinal microvascular abnormalities (IRMA). These warning signs may herald the appearance of the retinal or optic discs new vessels, which should not be confused with normal disc capillaries or with

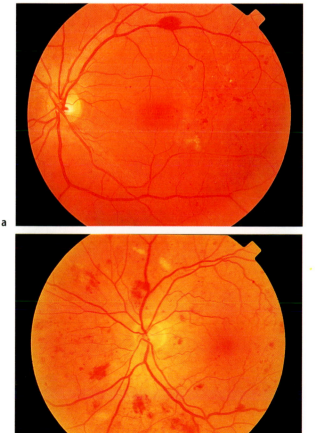

Fig. 21.2. Background diabetic retinopathy. **a** Early: microaneurysms and haemorrhages. **b** Severe: extensive haemorrhages, cotton-wool spots and venous dilatation.

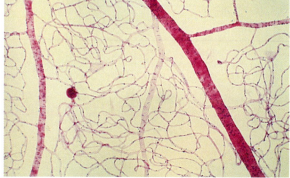

Fig. 21.3. Trypsin digest of retina showing microaneursyms and loss of some mural cells.

widened collateral vessels. Approximately 50% of eyes with preproliferative changes will progress to proliferative disease within one year.

Proliferative Retinopathy

Proliferative diabetic retinopathy (PDR) occurs in 5% of all diabetics. Younger onset diabetics have an increased risk of PDR after 30 years. Until recently 50–70% of PDR cases became blind within five years.

PDR is characterised by the development of new blood vessels (neovascularisation) on the optic nerve head or the retina (Figure 21.4). These occur as a response to retinal ischaemia. These new vessels may appear as small tufts, which ramify irregularly. They may be flat initially but enlarge and move forwards into the vitreous cavity as they grow. Once the new vessels form and grow, there is increased risk of an acute pre-retinal or vitreous haemorrhage. This is a significant threat to vision because the vitreous haemorrhages may become recurrent or dense preventing any meaningful examination and treatment. Retinal fibrosis, traction retinal detachment and neovascular glaucoma may occur at a later stage.

It is important to appreciate that proliferative retinopathy may be quite severe before the patient notices anything and the situation may have to be explained very carefully to him or her.

Diabetic Maculopathy

This is the commonest cause of visual impairment in diabetics. It occurs more commonly in type II diabetics. Three types of maculopathy are known and these may occur in isolation or in combination with each other. The three types are:

● Focal due to focal leakage from a microaneurysm or dilated capillaries and surrounding exudates are seen (Figure 21.5).
● Diffuse oedema caused by diffuse leakage from dilated capillaries at the posterior pole of the eye. Retinal oedema is diffuse and may be associated with microaneurysms and few haemorrhages but exudates are absent (Figure 21.6).
● Ischaemic maculopathy is due to closure of the perifoveal and surrounding vascular network. In addition to diffuse oedema several dark haemorrhages may be present (Figure 21.7). Fluorescein angiography may be required to confirm the ischaemia and determine its severity (Figure 21.7).

Treatment

Control of Diabetes

This aspect of treatment may seem self-evident but in the past the value of careful control has not always been fully recognised. Some patents have the impression that eye problems develop anyway if the diabetes has been present long enough. Nothing

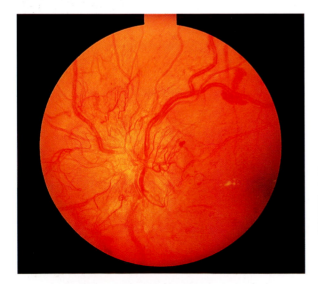

Fig. 21.4. Proliferative diabetic retinopathy.

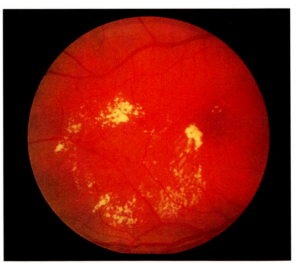

Fig. 21.5. Focal maculopathy.

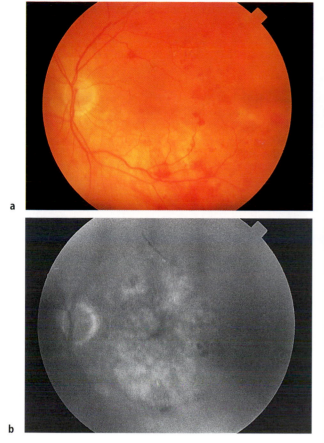

Fig. 21.6. Macular oedema: **a** colour photograph; **b** fluorescein angiogram of eye in **a** showing diffuse and cystoid oedema.

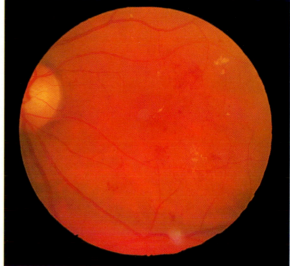

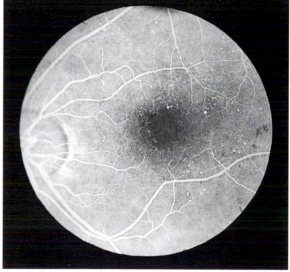

Fig. 21.7. Ischaemic maculopathy: **a** colour photograph; **b** fluorescein angiogram.

could be further from the truth. Control of the diabetic state needs to be sustained.

Laser Photocoagulation

The use of a focused light beam to cauterise the retina has been practised for several years and the value of this treatment has been confirmed by extensive clinical trials for both proliferative disease and some types of maculopathy. The exact mode of action is not known but it has been suggested that the photocoagulation of ischaemic areas prevents the release of some, as yet unidentified, vasoformative factor in proliferative disease. The treatment must be applied promptly in the early proliferative stage or sometimes before. About 2500–3000 burns (of 500 m spot size) are needed in an eye with proliferative retinopathy. This may require several treatment sessions (Figure 21.8). The laser treatment of

focal and diffuse maculopathy involves application of small number of burns (of 100–200 μm spot size) to the leaking area, avoiding the fovea. Ischaemic maculopathy generally is less amenable to laser treatment.

Glaucoma Surgery

Drainage surgery may be needed if neovascular glaucoma is not controlled by medical means. Rubeosis iridis initially requires panretinal laser

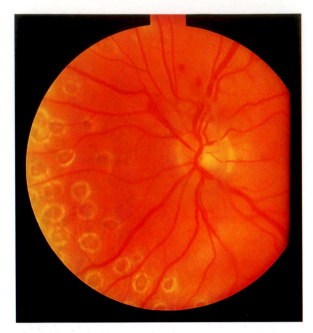

Fig. 21.8. Panretinal laser photocoagulation in proliferative diabetic retinopathy.

photocoagulation. Chronic simple glaucoma may also be more common in diabetics. Drainage surgery in these cases is less successful than in non-diabetics. Special measures need to be taken to avoid failure.

Vitreo-retinal Surgery

There have been dramatic advances in the technical side of vitreous surgery in recent years so that it is now possible to remove a persistent vitreous haemorrhage and to divide or remove fibrous tissue, even from the surface of the retina and relieve traction retinal detachment. Vitrectomy for vitreous haemorrhage tends to be performed sooner these days because of the relative safety of the technique. It may be combined with intraoperative laser photocoagulation.

Prognosis

A better understanding of diabetic retinopathy has resulted from the use of more accurate methods of investigation, especially fluorescein angiography and also the routine use of indirect ophthalmoscopy and slit-lamp microscopy. Serial fundus photography and the use of ultrasound have also been important. This better understanding and modern technology have led to more effective treatment so that the more severe ocular complications are now largely avoidable. Blindness tends to be limited to those cases where social or other circumstances make management difficult. Patient education is essential in order to maintain continuing improvement in visual prognosis for diabetics. Seventy-five per cent of diabetics will develop some form of retinopathy after 20 years. About 70% of patients with proliferative retinopathy will progress to blindness if untreated in five years.

Thyroid Eye Disease

Dysthyroid eye disease is an autoimmune disease in which the manifestations may be notable in the hyperthyroid, euthyroid or hypothyroid phase. Although the ophthalmic features of thyroid disease are often diagnosed in the hyperthyroid phase, a significant number of patients may be euthyroid (i.e. have no other evidence of thyroid disease) or less often hypothyroid at the time of detection of the eye changes. Thus the ophthalmic disease may precede, be coincidental or follow the systemic manifestations.

Graves' disease is a term used to describe the most common form of hyperthyroidism that has an autoimmune basis. Hyperthyroidism may arise from other conditions, for excample, thyroid tumour or pituitary dysfunction. It usually affects women between 20 and 45 years. Usually it is characterised by goitre, infiltrative ophthalmopathy, thyroid acropathy (clubbing) and pretibial myxoedema. When these ophthalmic changes occur in isolation the condition is described as ophthalmic Graves' disease (OGD).

The systemic features of hyperthyroidism include weight loss, high pulse rate, poor tolerance of warm weather and fine tremor. The eye signs of thyroid disease are eyelid retraction and lid lag, puffiness of the eyelids, chemosis, proptosis, exposure keratitis, double vision from muscle involvement and optic neuropathy (see Tables 21.2 and 21.3):

● *Lid retraction.* Eyelid drawn up slightly, more on one side than the other. Reveals white sclera above corneoscleral junction (Figure 21.9).
● *Lid lag.* When instructed to follow a pencil as it moves downwards, the upper lid appears to lag behind the rotation of the eye, revealing more of the white above. The upper lid shows jerky movements as the eye rotates smoothly down.

Table 21.2. The 13 possible eye signs of thyroid disease

- Proptosis
- Raised intraocular pressure when looking up
- Lid lag
- Lid retraction
- Lid swelling
- Chemosis
- Conjunctival congestion
- Extraocular muscle limitation
- Exposure keratitis
- Corneal ulceration
- Optic disc swelling
- Impaired visual acuity
- Constriction of visual field

Table 21.3. Routine tests for thyrotoxicosis

- Serum thyroxine (T4)
- Thyroid autoantibodies
- T3 assay

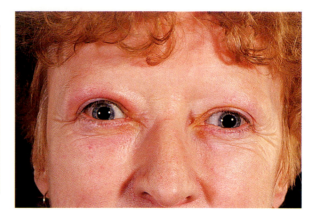

Fig. 21.10. Dysthyroid eye disease: lid oedema.

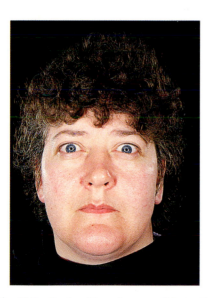

Fig. 21.9. Dysthyroid eye disease: eyelid retraction.

● *Lid swelling*. Puffiness of the eyelids may be present (Figure 21.10).

● *Chemosis*. This means conjunctival oedema. To the naked eye it appears as though the eyes are brimming with tears, and the expression "the tear that never drops" is sometimes used. When severe, the conjunctiva overhangs the lower lid margin.

● *Proptosis*. Lid retraction may give the false impression of proptosis but measurement of the position of the globe in relation to the bony orbit can be achieved by means of an exophthalmometer. Any relative protrusion can thus be measured for future reference. Dysthyroid disease is the commonest cause of unilateral or bilateral proptosis. Forward protrusion of the globe may lead to severe exposure keratitis demanding urgent attention.

● *Exposure keratitis*. Punctate staining with fluorescein across the lower part of the cornea is characteristic and due to inadequate closure of the retracted upper lid.

● *Limitation of extraocular muscle action*. The muscles become infiltrated and thickened producing a characteristic appearance on CT scan, which helps to distinguish this form from other causes of diplopia. The main restriction of movement is due to infiltration then subsequently tethering of the inferior recti with limitation of upward gaze. The resulting pressure on the globe may cause the intraocular pressure to rise on looking up and this has been used as a diagnostic test. The other extraocular muscles are involved less frequently.

● *Optic nerve compression*. This condition occurs only in 5% of cases of thyroid eye disease. However, it is important because of the seriousness of the condition. It is due to the increased pressure within the orbit, where enlargement of the extraocular muscle causes crowding of the orbital apex with subsequent compression of the optic nerve. The first sign may be swelling of the optic disc, followed by optic atrophy. It is therefore very important to monitor the visual acuity and central visual field in these cases.

Management

Reassurance is all that may be required in the mild forms of the disease. In some cases treatment is usually limited to that of the exposure keratitis. Ocular lubrication with artificial tear drops, and an antibiotic ointment instilled at night is often sufficient. Sometimes a small lateral tarsorrhaphy on each side can greatly improve the appearance of a young girl with lid retraction. Lid retraction may also be improved by the use of guanethidine eyedrops.

If there is visual deterioration (from optic nerve compression or significant proptosis) large doses of systemic steroids are probably the best line of treatment (e.g. prednisolone 120 mg/day). Initial recovery is usually dramatic and rapid but then the side-effects of systemic steroids ensue. The dose should be reduced as soon as feasible but it may be necessary to continue with a maintenance dose for many months. Some ophthalmolgists may use other immunosuppressive agents, for example, azathioprine or orbital radiotherapy in severe cases of proptosis and or optic nerve compression. If there is no response between 24–48 h, surgical decompression of the orbits is required. If double vision persists beyond the acute stage, extraocular muscle surgery may be helpful and operations have also been designed to deal with lid retraction.

Hypertension

Although the effects of raised blood pressure on the appearance of the fundus of the eye were recognised in the nineteenth century, the nature of the detailed changes is still disputed. Certain characteristic features, such as the nipping of the veins at arteriovenous crossings, narrowing of the arterioles, haemorrhages, papilloedema and exudates, are beyond doubt. Some confusion can be avoided if it is realised that the effects of raised blood pressure are modified by other changes in the eye due to natural ageing. It is now accepted that the exact cause of the raised blood pressure does not by itself influence the fundus appearance. However the appearance of the retinal vessels and associated changes serve as a good guide to the severity of the disease and urgency of treatment.

The Effect of Age on the Retinal Blood Vessels

In older patients the retinal arteries are seen to be narrower and straighter and the veins are also narrower than in younger patients. The term "retinal arteriosclerosis" is used to describe these changes.

The Effects of Raised Blood Pressure on the Retinal Vessels

In younger patients, irregular narrowing of the retinal arterioles is seen, and is thought by many to be due to spasm of the vessel walls. This hypertonicity leads in time to more permanent changes in the vessel walls so that the vessels resemble those of an older patient. Nipping of the veins at arteriovenous crossings is seen and on the distal side of the crossing the vein may be distended. Occasional flame haemorrhages, cotton-wool spots and exudates, may indicate more severe vascular damage but do not necessarily lead to "malignant" hypertension (Figure 21.11).

In older patients, the already narrowed vessels tend to show less dramatic changes. Hypertonicity of the vessel walls is not seen but arteriovenous nipping remains an important sign and haemorrhages may be present in more severe cases. The cotton-wool spots of hypertension reflect ischaemic damage to the nerve fibre layer due to obstruction of the retinal pre-capillary arterioles. Exudates are due to abnormal vascular permeability.

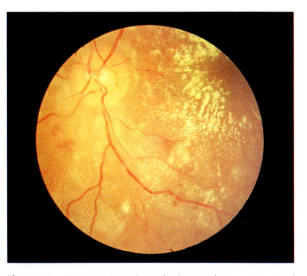

Fig. 21.11. Hypertensive retinopathy: haemorrhages, cotton-wool spots, exudates, vascular calibre changes.

"Malignant" Hypertension

Occasionally patients with a severe hypertensive problem present directly to the ophthalmologist because their main symptom is blurring of the vision, the other more usual symptoms being less evident. On examination, the visual acuity may be only slightly reduced unless there is significant macular oedema and there may be some enlargement of the blind spot and constriction of the visual fields. Inspection of the fundus reveals marked swelling of the optic disc, the oedema often extending well away from the disc with scattered flame-shaped haemorrhages. If the diastolic blood pressure is above 110–120 mmHg, there is little doubt about the diagnosis, but below this level it is essential to bear in mind the possibility of raised intracranial pressure from other causes. When hypertension is as severe as this the patient should be treated as an acute medical emergency and referred without delay to the appropriate physician.

Other Associated Vascular Changes

Retinal vascular Occlusion

This is more common in hypertensive patients compared to normotensives. The most frequent occurrence is the central retinal vein occlusion (CRVO) although branch retinal vein occlusion (BRVO) may occur at arterio-venous crossings. The fundus appearance in CRVO is dramatic with numerous scattered haemorrhages and swelling of the optic disc and the patient experiences sudden blurring of vision in one eye (Figure 21.12). This can be compared with occlusion of the central retinal artery which is less common and in which the prognosis is uniformly worse. Here the fundus appears pale and the arteries are narrowed. There is a cherry-red spot at the macula.

Emboli

Cholesterol emboli may be seen in the retinal arteries, sometimes in association with arterial occlusion. These usually arise from atheromatous plaques in the carotid artery. Calcified emboli may be seen in association with diseased heart valves and platelet or fibrin emboli may also be observed.

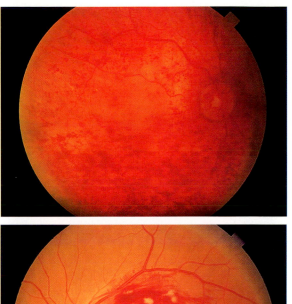
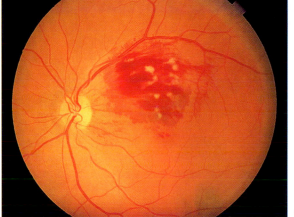

Fig. 21.12.   **a** Central retinal vein occlusion and **b** macular branch retinal vein occlusion.

Ischaemic Optic Neuropathy

Some elderly patients complaining of visual loss in one eye are found to have a pale swollen optic disc and sometimes evidence of branch retinal artery occlusion, giving an altitudinal defect of the visual field. This appearance should suggest the possibility of temporal arteritis and an ESR and a temporal artery biopsy should be considered as urgent investigations (Figure 21.13).

However, there is a group known as "non-arteritic" or idiopathic anterior ischaemic optic neuropathy (AION) which occurs in otherwise healthy individuals between 45 and 65 years of age,. About one-third of these patients develop bilateral disease. In these patients retinal arterial occlusion is absent. There is no known treatment for non-arteritic AION but giant cell arteritis needs exclusion.

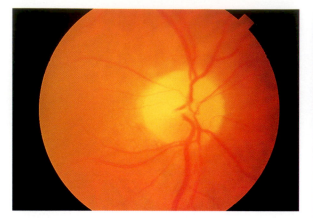

Fig. 21.13.   Anterior ischaemic optic neuropathy. The superior part of the disc is pale.

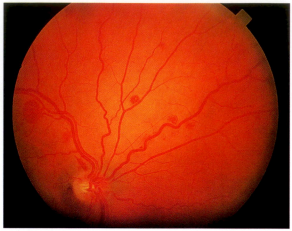

Fig. 21.14.   The fundus in leukaemia. Note dilated veins and haemorrhages.

Anaemia

When the haemoglobin concentration in the blood is abnormally low, this becomes apparent in the conjunctiva and ocular fundus. The conjunctiva, similar to oral mucosa is pale. The retinal vessels become pale and the difference between arteries and veins becomes less apparent. The fundus background also appears pale but this sign is dependent on the natural pigmentation of the fundus and may be misleading. In severe cases small haemorrhages are usually seen, mainly around the optic disc. The haemorrhages tend to be flame-shaped but a special feature of anaemic retinopathy is the presence of white areas in the centre of some of the haemorrhages. The haemorrhages may be due to associated low platelet counts. In pernicious anaemia, retinal haemorrhages and bilateral optic neuropathy which manifests as centrocaecal scotomas are seen.

In severe cases the optic nerves are atrophic. Anaemia secondary to blood loss may give rise to ocular hypoperfusion, which leads to anterior ischaemic optic neuropathy. Examination of the conjunctiva is perhaps of more value – or at least is certainly an easier way of assessing the haemoglobin level – and this part of the examination of the eye should, of course, precede ophthalmoscopy.

The Leukaemias

All ocular tissue may be involved in leukaemia. The eye changes may occur at any time during the course of leukaemia, or they may comprise the presenting features of the disease. These changes are more common in the acute leukaemias than in the chronic types.

Two groups of ophthalmic manifestations are recognised in leukaemias. The first group consists of leukaemic infiltration of ocular structures for example, retinal and pre-retinal infiltrates or anterior chamber and iris deposits. All of these are quite uncommon. The second group of manifestations is considered to be secondary to the haematological changes for example, thrombocytopenia, increased blood viscosity and highly increased leucocyte count. These changes include subconjunctival haemorrhages, intraretinal haemorrhages including white centred ones, cotton-wool spots, "slow flow retinopathy" (Figure 21.14) and retinal venous occlusions (especially CRVO).

Less common manifestations include choroidal infiltrations, retinal and optic disc neovascularisations. Apart from eye changes, the vision may be impaired by leukaemic infiltrates elsewhere in the visual pathway (leading to field defects).

Ocular disease may also occur as complications of treatment of the leukaemia, for example, opportunistic infections such as herpes zoster, graft-versus-host reactions and intraocular haemorrhage.

Sickle-cell Disease

This condition is mentioned separately because of the severe and devastating effect it may have on the vision. The sickle-cell haemoglobinopathies are inherited and are due to the affected person having one or more abnormal haemoglobins as recognised by the electrophoretic pattern and labelled alphabetically. Haemoglobins S and C are the most important ophthalmologically. Thalassaemia (persistence of fetal haemoglobin) can also cause retinopathy. The abnormal haemoglobins occur either in combination with normal haemoglobins resulting in AS (sickle-cell trait) or in association with each other SS (sickle-cell anaemia or disease) or SC (sickle-cell haemoglobin C disease) and S thal (thalassemia). Individuals with cell trait usually lead a normal life and do not have any systemic or ocular complications. The red blood cells in patients with sickle-cell (SS, SC, S thal) disease adopt abnormal shapes under hypoxia and acidosis. These abnormal red cells are less deformable compared to normal and leads to occlusion of the small retinal blood vessels especially in the retinal periphery.

Sickle-cell retinopathy can be divided into two types: non-proliferative and proliferative. In non-proliferative sickle retinopathy there is increased venous tortuosity, peripheral chorioretinal atrophy, peripheral retinal haemorrhages, peripheral haemosiderin deposits which appear refractile, and peripheral arterial occlusion. These lesions are usually asymptomatic. When central retinal, arterial or venous occlusion, macular arteriolar occlusion or choroidal ischaemia occur there is significant visual deficit.

When significant ischaemia is present retinal neovascularisation occurs. This is generally in the retinal periphery. Such peripheral neovascularisation may respond to laser photocoagulation or cryotherapy of the retina. Occasionally vitrectomy is required.

Onchocerciasis

Onchocerciasis, commonly known as river blindess, is caused by the filaria onchocerca volvulus. The name "river blindness" is derived from the occurrence of the disease in focal areas along rivers and streams where the blackfly (Similium) breeds in fast-flowing water. The blackfly can travel several kilometres and does not respect international borders.

The disease is characterised by a few adult worms encased in nodules and the invasion of the body by microfilaria. It is endemic in equatorial Africa – west and central and South America. It is estimated that

there are about half a million blind people due to onchocerciasis.

The adult worm has a lifespan of 15–30 years. The microfilaria is sucked up by the blackfly when it takes its blood meal. Subsequently, division within the blackfly gives rise to latter stages of the larva, which are re-injected, into the skin of the next vicim of the blackfly's bite. The microfilariae migrate under and through the skin and may mature in about one year. Newly produced microfilariae migrate to the eye through the skin or blood.

Clinical manifestations of onchocerciasis may be divided into extraocular and ocular manifestations.

- *Extraocular features*
  - skin; pruritis – a maculopapular rash, which may be associated with hypopigmentation or hyperpigmentation, dermal, and epidermal atrophy or "onchodermatitis"
  - subcutaneous nodules – which are firm, round masses in the dermis and subcutaneous tissue, especially close to joints in the head and shoulder.
- *Ocular features*
  - intraocular microfilariae may be seen in the anterior chamber. Dead microfilaria are usually seen in the cornea (especially peripherally)
  - punctate keratitis and sclerosing keratitis
  - anterior uveitis, usually of the non-granulomatous type with loss of the pigment frill, and posterior synechiae are common. Secondary cataract and glaucoma may develop
  - chorioretinitis of the chronic non-granulomatous type with secondary degenerative changes in the RPE neuroretina and the choriocapillaries. There may be granular atrophy of the RPE, subretinal fibrosis, retinal arteriolar attenuation and vasculitis. Optic atrophy and neuropathy are not uncommon.

Diagnosis is confirmed by skin snip and the Mazzoti test which depends on a Herxheimer reaction to a single dose of diethylcarbamazine (DECM). Care is required with this test since the reaction could be very severe.

Management

Management is by vector control and chemotherapy. Presently an international (World Health Organization) programme, the Onchocerciasis Control

Programme (OCP), is underway in the Volta River Basin. Chemotherapy of infected patients now uses Ivermectin, which in a single dose rids the patient of microfilaria for one to two years. This medication needs to be repeated over several years in mass administration projects.

Diethylcarbamazine is the older treatment for the microfilaria but is more toxic and requires to be taken over a 2–3-week period. Adult worms can only be killed by suramin, or removed surgically.

Acquired Immune Deficiency Syndrome (AIDS)

AIDS refers to the final stages of infection by the human immunodeficiency virus (HIV). The earlier stages of the disease are often asymptomatic (Table 21.4).

In western countries, AIDS commonly affects homosexuals, haemophiliacs, and intravenous drug abusers, although there is now a significant heterosexual and paediatric pool of patients. In Africa, it is generally a heterosexual disease, and a significant paediatric population is also known. Transmission is through sexual intercourse, parenteral or transplacental routes.

Ocular features occur in 75% of patients with AIDS. The major ocular complications of AIDS occur later in the disease and can be predicted by CD4 T cell levels. At CD4 level > 200×10^6/L common ocular complications are toxoplasmosis and herpes zoster ophthalmicus and retinitis whilst at CD4 levels < 50×10^6/L cytomegalovirus (CMV) retinitis is common (Figure 21.15).

AIDS microangiopathy (non-infectious) occurs in about 50% of patients (in both developing and

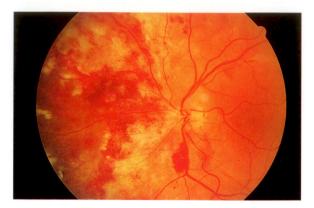

Fig. 21.15. Cytomegalovirus retinitis in acquired immune deficiency syndrome.

western countries). It consists of microaneurysms, telangiectasia cotton-wool spots and a few retinal haemorrhages (Figure 21.16). Retinal peripheral perivascular sheathing may sometimes occur in the absence of intraocular infections.

Other ocular involvement of AIDS includes infections with opportunistic and non-opportunistic organisms (e.g. CMV, *Cryptococcus contagiosum*). Neoplasms of the conjunctiva, lids and orbit, and neuroophthalmic complications are other features.

In western countries, the commonest ophthalmic complications of AIDS is CMV retinitis whilst in developing countries (such as Africa), CMV is not a major problem; Herpes zoster ophthalmicus and conjunctival carcinoma are common in AIDS patients in Africa and AIDS patients die of other complications, for example, tuberculosis. Therefore short-term survival from AIDS itself is a problem in

Table 21.4. Classification of human immunodeficiency virus infection (Centers for Disease Control, Atlanta, 1992)

Group I	Acute infection: asymptomatic with seroconversion
Group II	Asymptomatic carrier
Group III	Generalised, persistent lymphadenopathies; usually good state of general health
Group IV AIDS Sub-groups	(A) Constitutional (cachexia, fever, etc.). (B) Neurological. (C) Infections diagnostic of AIDS. (D) Malignancies. (E) Others, e.g. CD4 counts < 200×10^6/L.

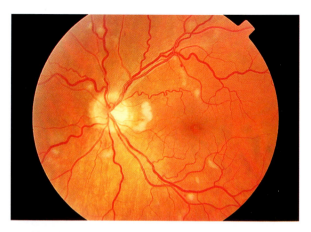

Fig. 21.16. Human immunodeficiency virus retinopathy.

developing countries while in western countries quality of life for the longer term is the main problem.

Ophthalmological Signs of AIDS

1. Non-infectious retinopathy:
   - cotton-wool spots
   - retinal haemorrhages
   - microvascular changes.
2. Opportunistic infections:
   - involvement of posterior segment
     - CMV retinitis
     - acute retinal necrosis (herpes simplex, zoster)
     - toxoplasmic chorioretinitis
     - *Pneumocystis carinii* choroiditis
     - tuberculous choroiditis
     - endophthalmitis caused by *Candida albicans* – usually in intravenous drug users
     - *Cryptococcus chorioretinitis*
     - syphilitic retinitis
   - involvement of anterior segment
     - chronic keratitis and keratouveitis caused by herpes zoster and simplex keratoconjunctivitis caused by CMV, microsporum and gonococcus
     - corneal ulcer caused by *C. albicans* and bacteria (*Pseudomonas aeruginosa*, *Staphylococcus aureus* and *S. epidermidis*)
     - syphilitic and toxoplasmic iridocyclitis
     - conjunctivitis caused by CMV, herpes zoster and simplex
     - bacterial conjunctivitis.
3. Neoplasms:
   - conjunctival, palpebral and orbital Kaposi's sarcoma
   - intraocular lymphoma
   - other neoplasms
     - conjunctival squamous carcinoma
     - palpebral and orbital lymphoma.

4. Neuro-ophthalmological signs:
   - involvement of cranial nerves
     - internuclear ophthalmoplegia
     - IIIrd, IVth and VIth cranial nerve palsies
     - retrobulbar neuritis and papillitis
   - homonymous hemianopia
   - AIDS–dementia complex with cortical blindness.

5. Other signs:
   - conjunctiva
     - non-specific conjunctivitis
     - keratoconjunctivitis sicca
     - non-specific conjunctiva microvascular changes in the inferior perilimbal bulbar region (haemorrhages, microaneurysms, column fragmentation, dilatation, and irregular vessel diameter)
     - bacterial conjunctivitis
   - cornea
     - non-specific punctate keratitis
   - sclera
     - necrotising scleritis
   - retina
     - talc-induced retinopathy (only intravenous drug users)
   - eyelids
     - herpes zoster ophthalmicus
     - palpebral molluscum contagiosum
     - palpebral cryptococcosis
   - orbit
     - orbital apex granuloma
     - orbital pseudotumour
     - orbital infiltration by *Aspergillus*, *Pneumocystis carinii*
     - orbital cellulitis
   - visual and refraction defects
     - night blindness due to vitamin A and E malabsorption
     - progression of myopia
     - decreased accommodation
   - acute closed angle (bilateral) glaucoma caused by choroidal effusion.

Neuro-ophthalmology 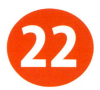 **22**

It is found in most ophthalmic departments that it is necessary to retain a close liaison with neurological and neurosurgical departments, and neuro-ophthalmology is now in itself a subspecialty. Retrobulbar neuritis, for example, is a condition, which presents quite commonly to eye casualty departments and usually requires further investigation by a neurologist. Less common, but equally important are the pituitary tumours which, it will be seen, can present in a subtle way to the ophthalmologist and which may require urgent medical attention. There are many other, sometimes rare, conditions, which find common ground between the disciplines.

The Optic Disc

Normal Disc

One must be familiar with some of the variations found in otherwise normal individuals before being able to diagnose pathological changes. The optic discs mark the entrance of the optic nerves to the eye and this small circular part of the fundus is non-seeing and corresponds with blind spots in the visual field. When examining an optic disc, five important features are to be noted:

- colour
- margins or contour
- vessel entry
- central cup
- presence or absence of haemorrhages.

Colour

The disc is pink but often slightly paler on the temporal side. That of the neonate may be deceptively pale and some elderly discs appear atrophic without evidence of disease. Pallor of the disc is due to loss of nerve tissue and small blood vessels of the disc. In very severe optic atrophic cupping, there is exposure of the underlying sclera. The myopic disc is relatively pale, whereas the hypermetropic disc is pinker than normal (Figure 22.1).

Margins

These are better defined in myopic than in hypermetropic subjects. In hypermetropes the edges of the disc may appear raised, sometimes resembling papilloedema. It is common to see a crescent of pigment on the temporal side of the disc. However the presence of chorioretinal atrophy at the disc margin in myopes may give rise to difficulty in deciding where the true disc margin is.

Vessel Entry

In general, a central retinal artery and vein divide into upper and lower branches which in turn divide into nasal and temporal branches close to the disc margin. Many variations in the pattern are seen normally. The veins are darker and wider than the arteries and, unlike the arteries, can be seen to pulsate spontaneously in 80% of the population if examined carefully. In the other 20% normals, venous pulsation at the disc can be induced by gentle pressure on the globe.

Central Cup

The centre of the disc is deeper, for instance, further away from the observer, than the peripheral part. This central cup occupies about one-third (or less) of the total disc diameter in normal subjects. The ratio between the vertical diameter of the cup

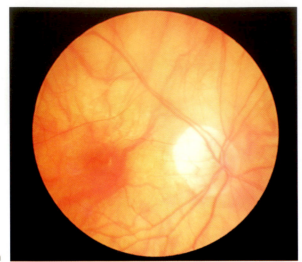

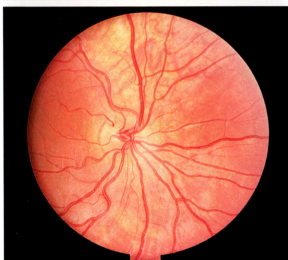

Fig. 22.1.   Normal optic disc in **a** myope and **b** hypermetrope.

compared to disc diameter is known as the cup-to-disc ratio. Thus the normal cup-to-disc ratio is < 0.3.

Haemorrhages

Haemorrhages are never seen on or adjacent to normal discs.

Congenital Disc Anomalies

A number of minor congenital abnormalities are seen on the disc. In an astigmatic eye the disc is often oval. The central cup may be filled in by "drusen" – small hyaline deposits, which may be found on the surface or buried in the substance of the disc. Alternatively, the central cup may be hollowed out further by a congenital pit in the disc. Myelinated nerve fibres are recognised by their strikingly white appearance, which obscures any underlying vessels, and their fluffy margin. The central cup may be filled in by persistent remnants of the hyaloid artery, which runs in the embryo from disc to lens. Some of these and other congenital abnormalities of the disc may be associated with visual field defects which are not progressive but which can cause diagnostic confusion.

Pale Disc

Optic Atrophy

Optic atrophy means loss of nerve tissue on the disc, and the resulting abnormal pallor of the disc must be accompanied by a defect in the visual field, but not necessarily by a reduction in the visual acuity. It must be remembered that the disc tends to be somewhat pale and the cup of disc tends to be larger in short-sighted eyes and care must be taken in diagnosing optic atrophy in such cases. The number of small vessels, which can be counted on the disc, is sometimes used as an index of atrophy in difficult cases.

Classification of the causes of optic atrophy usually includes the term "consecutive optic atrophy", referring to atrophy following retinal degeneration. The terms primary and secondary atrophy are also used but because these terms are confusing a simple aetiological classification will be used here. It should be borne in mind that it is not usually possible to determine the cause of optic atrophy by the appearance of the optic disc. Even the cupped, pale disc of chronic glaucoma may be mimicked by optic atrophy due to chiasmal compression. When optic atrophy follows swelling of the optic disc, there is more gliosis than when it is "primary", that is, due to disease in the nerve itself. Gliosis makes the appearance of the disc more grey or yellowish-grey than white and the cribriform markings often seen in optic atrophy may not be evident.

The following are the important causes of optic atrophy:

● Glaucoma.

● Vascular. Following obstruction of the central retinal artery or vein, and anterior ischaemic optic neuropathy.

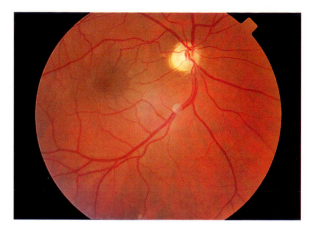

Fig. 22.2. Optic atrophy due to pituitary compression of optic nerve.

● Following disease in the optic nerve, for example, optic neuritis or compression of the nerve by an aneurysm or tumour (Figure 22.2).

● Following papilloedema: the disc may become atrophic as a direct result of the chronic swelling, irrespective of its cause.

● Inherited. Retinitis pigmentosa is an inherited retinal degeneration in which there is a progressive night blindness, constriction of the visual field and scattered pigmentation in the fundus. As the condition advances towards blindness, the discs become atrophic. Optic atrophy may also appear in certain families without any other apparent pathology, for example, Leber's optic atrophy and congenital or infantile optic atrophy. It is also seen in the rare but distressing cerebro-retinal degenerations, which presents with progressive blindness, epilepsy and dementia.

● Toxic. A number of poisons can specifically damage the optic nerve; methanol is a classical example. Tobacco amblyopia is a type of progressive atrophy due to excessive smoking of coarse tobacco, usually in a pipe and often in association with a high ethanol intake. Reversal may be achieved by abstention in the early phases of the disease.

● Trauma. The optic nerve may be damaged by indirect injury if bleeding occurs into the dural sheath. This may result from a fracture in the region of the optic foramen or rarely, from contusion of the eye itself. After the nerve has been damaged, a period of a few weeks elapses before the nerve head becomes atrophic, so that initially the eye may be blind but the fundus normal. The pupil reaction to direct light is impaired from the time of the injury.

Such an injury may result in complete and permanent blindness in the affected eye but a degree of recovery is achieved in a small proportion of cases, if decompression of the nerve sheath is undertaken early.

Swelling of the Optic Disc

This is a serious sign because it may be due to raised intracranial pressure and an intracranial space-occupying lesion. There are, however, a number of other more common causes.

Apparent Swelling

The margins of the optic disc may be ill-defined and even appear swollen in hypermetropic eyes. Other congenital abnormalities of the disc such as drusen or myelination of the nerve fibres may also be mistaken for true swelling (Figure 22.3).

Vascular

The disc may be swollen in congestive cardiac failure or in patients with severe chronic emphysema. Marked swelling of the disc with numerous haemorrhages is seen in occlusion of the central retinal vein and this compares with the pale and less haemorrhagic swelling that is seen in ischaemic optic neuropathy. In the latter instance, swelling of the disc occurs in association with arterial disease and

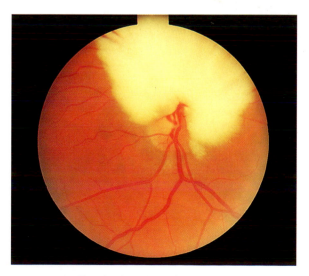

Fig. 22.3. Myelinated nerve fibres.

one must take pains to exclude temporal arteritis in the elderly.

Postoperative

Swelling of the disc is not uncommon in the immediate postoperative period after intraocular surgery. It is due to ocular hypotony. It may persist for longer periods if the intraocular pressure remains low. It is not usually regarded to be of serious significance, since the swelling regresses following normalisation of the intraocular pressure.

True Papilloedema

Papilloedema is swelling of the optic discs due to increased intracranial pressure. Every doctor must be aware of the triad of headache, papilloedema and vomiting as an important feature of raised intracranial pressure. The optic disc may be markedly swollen and haemorrhages are present around it, but not usually in the peripheral fundus (Figure 22.4). In chronic papilloedema, the disc is paler and haemorrhages may be few or absent. Although these patients may complain of transient blurring of the vision, the visual acuity is usually normal and testing the visual fields shows only some enlargement of the blind spots. It is important to realise that the word "papilloedema" refers to the non-inflammatory swelling of the disc, which results from raised intracranial pressure. The most common causes of raised intracranial pressure are cerebral tumours, malignant hypertension, cerebral abscess, subdural haematoma, hydrocephalus and benign intracranial hypertension.

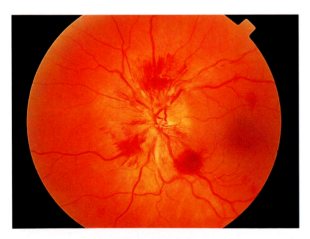

Fig. 22.4. Papilloedema.

Diagnosis of papilloedema entails careful examination of the optic disc, which must be backed up with visual field examination and colour fundus photography. The latter is especially helpful when repeated to show any change in the disc appearance. Fluorescein angiography may also be of great diagnostic help in difficult cases.

Optic Neuritis

This most commonly occurs in association with a plaque of demyelination in the optic nerve in patients with multiple sclerosis. The central vision is usually severely affected, in contrast with papilloedema, but optic neuritis occurs in many instances without any visible swelling of the disc.

Other Causes

Chronic intraocular inflammation such as anterior or intermediate uveitis may be complicated by disc swelling. Severe diabetic eye disease may sometimes be marked by disc swelling (diabetic papillopathy). In severe cases of thyrotoxic exophthalmos, the orbital congestion may cause disc swelling (dysthyroid optic neuropathy). In both instances the doctor should be warned that serious consequences might ensue unless prompt treatment is applied. Infiltration of the disc by leukaemia or lymphoma or chronic granulomata (as in sarcoidosis) may also cause disc swelling.

Multiple Sclerosis

This common and important neurological disease may often present initially as an eye problem and its proper management requires careful co-ordination at the primary care level. It is important to realise that multiple sclerosis should not be diagnosed after one single attack of retrobulbar neuritis since this could cause unnecessary alarm about something that may never happen. Furthermore, retrobulbar neuritis has causes other than multiple sclerosis. The diagnosis of multiple sclerosis should be made by a neurologist and is based on finding additional evidence of the disease elsewhere in the body.

The cause of multiple sclerosis is not known, but the disease is characterised by the appearance of multiple inflammatory foci in relation to the myelin sheaths of nerves throughout the central nervous system. The demyelination plaques are detectable on MRI scans of the brain. The optic nerve between globe and chiasm is commonly involved at an early stage and there may be a delay of several years before other features of the disease appear. Young or middle-aged people are mainly affected and the prognosis is worse when the disease is acquired at an early age.

Ocular Findings

Retrobulbar Neuritis

This is an important cause of unilateral sudden loss of vision in a white eye in a young person. The patient complains of pain behind the eye on attempting to move it and there is often a grey or coloured patch in the centre of the field of view. In severe cases the sight of the affected eye may be lost completely. On examination the pupil reaction is diminished on the affected side and this may be the only objective evidence of disease. It is essential to test the pupil before dilating it with eyedrops. The fundus is often normal initially, although there may be slight swelling of the optic disc. After two or three weeks the optic disc starts to become pale. The visual prognosis is generally good. Most patients make a complete or nearly complete recovery after six to twelve weeks. There is a risk, however, that the other eye may be affected at a later date and recurrent attacks in one or both eyes may cause permanent damage to the vision. Fortunately it is extremely rare for a patient to be made blind by multiple sclerosis. Papillitis in multiple sclerosis is uncommon and often occurs in children following viral infections.

The diagnosis at the time of the acute attack relies on the history and noting the pupil reaction. It is often advisable to make the diagnosis in retrospect. The patient may give a history of visual loss in one eye, which has recovered and at a later date presents with other non-ocular signs and symptoms of demyelinating disease. If it can be confirmed that the patient has had a previous attack of optic neuritis, this may help in the confirmation of the diagnosis of disseminated sclerosis. Under these circumstances the pallor of the disc may be helpful, but careful assessment of the colour vision, visual acuity and measurement of the visually evoked potential may provide conclusive evidence. At the time of the acute attack, testing the visual field may reveal a central scotoma. The size of this defect diminishes as healing occurs, often leaving a small residual defect between blind spot and central area.

Nystagmus

This usually appears at a later stage than optic neuritis and may only be evident in lateral gaze. It is often horizontal.

Internuclear Ophthalmoplegia

Whereas double vision is a common symptom in multiple sclerosis, it is unusual to see an obvious defect of the ocular movements. Sometimes it can be seen that one eye fails to turn inwards when the patient is asked to look to the opposite side, and yet when the patient is made to converge the eyes on a near object, the medial rectus moves normally. This failure of the muscle action with certain co-ordinated eye movements only, for instance, limitation of adduction, whilst the opposite abducting eye shows nystagmus is termed "internuclear ophthalmoplegia". It is very characteristic of multiple sclerosis when seen in young people (when the internuclear ophthalmoplegia is usually bilateral) but usually has a vascular cause in the elderly (when it is usually unilateral).

Other Features

Other types of ocular muscle dysfunction, for example, a lateral rectus palsy or ptosis, are rare. Careful inspection of the fundi in some cases reveals inflammatory changes around the retinal vessels especially in the periphery (peripheral retinal vasculitis).

Treatment conssists of corticosteroids administered systemically which may speed up recovery of vision. However, the final visual outcome is unchanged by such treatment.

Defects in the Visual Fields

The pattern of a visual field defect gives useful localising information for lesions in the visual pathway. The right half of each retina is linked by nerves to the right occipital cortex and the splitting of nerve fibres from each half occurs at the chiasm. For this reason lesions in the optic nerve anterior to the chiasm tend to cause unilateral defects whereas those posterior to the chiasm produce hemianopic or quadrantianopic defects (Figure 22.5). Cortical lesions tend to be more congruous. That is to say the blind areas on each side tend to be similar in shape and size. Cortical lesions also show better preservation of central vision ("macular sparing"). A

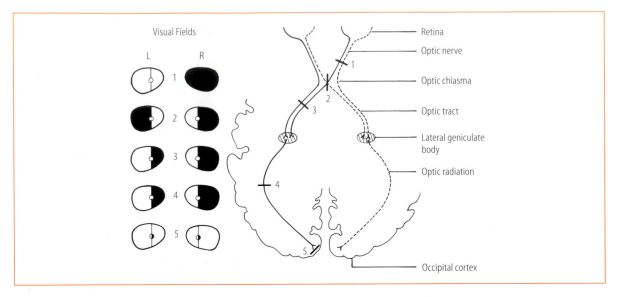

Fig. 22.5.   The visual pathway.

special type of field defect is seen with expanding pituitary tumours, the resulting pressure on the centre of the chiasm producing a bitemporal defect. Localised defects in the retina produce equivalent localised defects in the visual field on the affected side. Defects due to ocular disease are relatively common as for example those seen in the elderly with glaucoma. Care must be taken to interpret field defects with this possibility in mind. Notice from Figure 22.5 that the right half of the visual field is represented in the left half of each retina and thus the left half of the brain. This complies with the general rule that events occurring on the right side of the body are represented on the left side of the brain. It is surprising how patients may be unaware of a severe visual field defect, especially in hemianopia (Figure 22.6).

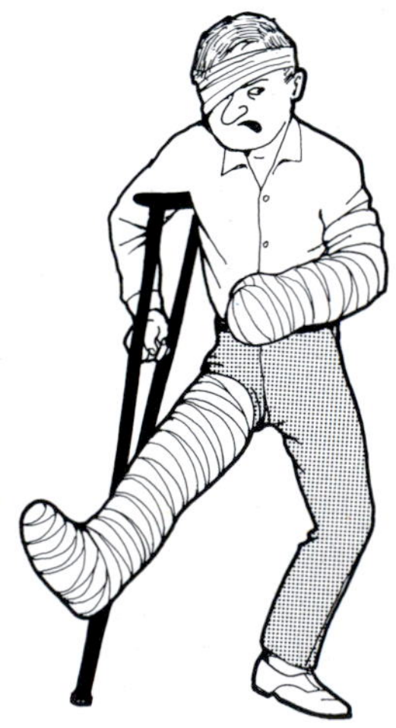

My car keeps knocking my gate post.
(Hemianopes should never drive)

Fig. 22.6.   The effects of hemianopia.

Abnormalities of the Pupil

The pupil constricts and dilates largely under the action of the sphincter muscle, which lines the pupil margin. It is supplied by parasympathetic fibres from the midbrain, which relay in the ciliary ganglion having been conveyed along the third cranial nerve (Figure 22.7). The dilator muscle is arranged radially within the iris and responds to the sympathetic nerves conveyed in the sympathetic plexus overlying the internal carotid artery. These fibres in turn arise from the superior cervical ganglion. The sympathetic supply to the dilator muscle therefore runs a long course from the hypothalamus to the midbrain and spinal cord and then up again from the root of the neck with the internal carotid artery.

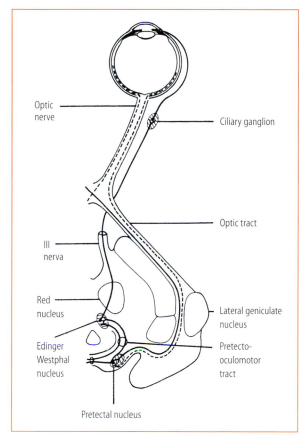

Optic
nerve

Ciliary ganglion

Optic tract

III
nerva

Red
nucleus

Lateral geniculate
nucleus

Edinger
Westphal
nucleus

Pretecto-
oculomotor
tract

Pretectal nucleus

Fig. 22.7. The pupillary pathway.

Miosis refers to a small pupil, mydriasis to a large pupil (big word, big pupil). The pupil grows smaller with age. In young children pupils are relatively large and sometimes anxious parents bring up their children because they are concerned about this. During sleep, the pupils become small. The pupils react to afferent stimuli conveyed along the optic nerves. The nerve fibres leave the optic tract without synapsing in the lateral geniculate nucleus. They pass to the pretectal nucleus of the midbrain where they synapse. When examining the eye with the ophthalmoscope it is evident that the pupil constricts more vigorously when the macula is examined than when the more peripheral fundus is stimulated with the ophthalmoscope light. When an eye is totally blind, usually there is no light pupil reaction but as a general rule, the pupils remain of equal size. It should be apparent from Figure 22.7 that the patient with cortical blindness may have a normal pupil reaction. We must also remember that a pupil may

not react to light because it is mechanically bound down to the lens by adhesions. When both maculae are damaged by senile macular degeneration, the pupils may be slightly wider than normal and may show sluggish reactions. An afferent pupil defect implies optic nerve or severe retinal disease.

The Abnormally Dilated Pupil

The most common reason for unilateral mydriasis is drugs in the form of locally administered eye drops, either prescribed by an ophthalmic department or obtained from a friend's medicine cabinet. The next most common cause is probably the Holmes–Adie's syndrome, a condition which is more common in young female patients.

The affected pupil is usually dilated and contracts very slowly in response to direct and indirect stimulation. In bright light the pupil may be constricted on the affected side and take some time to dilate in the dark. The pupillary constriction to near fixation is tonic and prolonged and worm-like. This tonic pupil reaction may be combined curiously with absent tendon jerks in the limbs. When the vision is blurred and the pupil widely dilated, the symptoms may be partially relieved by the use of a weak miotic. After a delay of months or years the other eye may become affected. The overall disability is minimal and the condition has not so far been related to any other systemic disease.

Acute narrow angle glaucoma can occasionally present in this manner and confusion may arise if the eye is not very red; however closer examination of the eye should make the diagnosis obvious. Since the nerve fibres, which cause constriction of the pupil, are conveyed in the oculomotor nerve, oculomotor palsy if complete is associated with mydriasis. For this reason dilatation of the pupil may be a serious sign of raised intracranial pressure after head injury. One pupil may be wider than the other as a congenital abnormality (congenital anisocoria).

The Abnormally Constricted Pupil

Again, drugs are a common cause. Miotic drops are still widely used for the treatment of chronic simple glaucoma and the constricted pupils of the morphine addict are well known if not so commonly seen. When a constricted pupil on one side is observed it is important to note the position of the eyelids. A slight degree of associated ptosis indicates the possibility of Horner's syndrome. The total syndrome comprises miosis, narrowing of the palpebral fissure due to paralysis of the smooth muscle in the eyelids (Müller's muscle), loss of sweating over the affected side of the forehead and a slight reduction of the intraocular pressure. Horner's syndrome may be caused by a wide diversity of lesions anywhere along the sympathetic pathway but quite often it is noted in the elderly as an isolated finding and investigation fails to reveal a cause. The Argyll Robertson (AR) pupil is a very rare but famous example of the miosed pupil, which responds to accommodation but not to direct light. This type of pupil reaction was originally described as being closely associated with syphilis of the central nervous system. The AR pupils show a more extensive reaction to near stimulation than light reflex. Visual acuity is normal in such patients.

Double Vision

Double vision (diplopia) may be monocular or binocular. Monocular diplopia, that is, diplopia that is still present when one eye is closed, is quite common and is usually due to cataract. Some patients say that they can see double when they mean that the vision is blurred. A clear distinction must therefore be made. Binocular double vision of recent onset should always be treated as a serious symptom. It is usually disabling, preventing the patient from working or even walking about. Some patients discover that the symptoms are relieved by placing a patch over one eye.

Slight degrees of double vision may be compensated by a head tilt or turn and the nature of the adopted head posture can help to identify the cause of the double vision. In the same way, if the history is elucidated carefully, noting, for example, whether the diplopia is worse for near or distance vision or whether there is horizontal or vertical displacement of the second image, then a possible cause may be suspected even before examining the patient.

Assessment of Eye Movements in Diplopia

The complaint of double vision suggests that the separate eyes are not both fixed on the point of regard. The eye that is "off-line" sees the object of regard but it appears displaced. This failure of the eyes to work together is due to malfunction of one or a group of eye muscles or the neurological mechanisms that control them.

From the clinical point of view it is convenient to divide the eye muscles into horizontal and vertical groups. The horizontal muscles, the medial and lateral recti, are easy to understand because their actions are in one plane and they simply adduct (turn in) or abduct (turn out) the globe. The vertical recti are best considered as having primary and secondary actions. It is important to realise that the action of the vertical recti changes with the position of the globe. For example, when the eye is abducted the superior rectus elevates the globe but when the eye is adducted the superior rectus rotates the eye inwards round an anterior–posterior axis (intorts). In a similar manner the inferior oblique elevates the adducted eye and extorts the abducted eye (Figure 22.8). In order to test the action of the superior oblique muscle, one must first ask the patient to adduct the eye and test for depression in adduction. That is to say a superior oblique palsy prevents the eye from looking down when it is turned in. The main line of action of the vertical recti is seen when the eye is abducted and that of the obliques is seen when the eye is adducted.

Examination of a patient with double vision entails first of all testing the gross eye movements in the cardinal positions of gaze and then noting the degree of separation of the images in these various positions. The Hess chart is one of several ingenious methods of recording the abnormal eye movements. The principle is to place a green filter before one eye and a red filter before the other and to ask the patient to look at a screen on which are placed a number of small illuminated white dots. The patient is then asked to

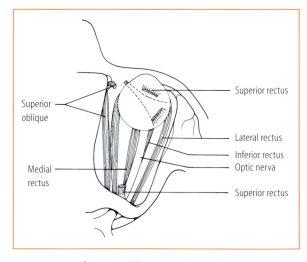

Fig. 22.8. The extraocular muscles.

localise the dots with a pointer. The amount of false localisation can then be measured in all positions of gaze. This technique is invaluable when assessing the recovery of an ocular muscle palsy.

Young children adapt to double vision very rapidly by suppressing the image from one eye, and under the age of eight years the suppression may lead to more permanent amblyopia if the situation is not relieved. In adults the double vision may persist and be disabling for months or even years if not treated by incorporating prisms into the spectacles or by muscle surgery.

Causes of Diplopia

● *Ocular muscle imbalance.* It will be recalled from the chapter on squint that some patients have a latent squint, which is controlled much of the time but sometimes becomes overt. A typical example is the hypermetrope with esophoria who begins to complain of double vision when working for an examination. This problem may be solved simply by prescribing suitable spectacles. Sometimes anxious patients who have had a squint since childhood begin to notice their double vision again, having suppressed one image for many years. The symptoms are usually relieved with the cause of the anxiety.

● *VIth cranial nerve palsy.* The affected eye is converged due to a weakness of the lateral rectus muscle. It occurs most commonly as an isolated episode in hypertensive elderly patients and heals spontaneously in 3–6 months. Elderly diabetics are also more prone to VIth cranial nerve palsies. In young patients the possibility of multiple sclerosis

or even raised intracranial pressure must be borne in mind.

● *IVth cranial nerve palsy.* The eye fails to look down when it is turned in and may be turned slightly up when the other eye is looking straight ahead. Trauma (a blow over the head) is an important cause in younger patients but a full investigation for an intracranial space-occupying lesion is usually needed.

● *IIIrd cranial nerve palsy.* The eye is turned out and slightly down, the pupil is dilated and ptosis is usually severe enough to close the eye. Trauma is an important cause is young people but carotid aneurysm and diabetes should also be considered.

● *Thyrotoxicosis.* Patients with this condition develop double vision because the extraocular muscles become infiltrated with inflammatory cells. The action of the inferior recti in particular becomes impaired and diplopia on upward gaze is a common sign.

● *Myasthenia gravis.* This disease presents sometimes with diplopia with or preceded by ptosis, which becomes worse as the day goes by. Any one muscle or group of muscles may be affected. The symptoms and signs show a transient improvement seconds after the intravenous injection of edrophonium chloride (Tensilon).

● *Blow-out fracture of the orbit.* A special cause of double vision following injury is the trapping of extraocular muscles, usually the inferior rectus in the line of fracture. The patient experiences double vision on looking upwards and the limitation of movement is evident. There may be a relative enophthalmos.

Genetics and the Eye 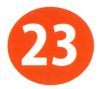 23

Several eye diseases are inherited or have familial clustering. It is therefore always advisable to enquire about the family history when interviewing a patient with ophthalmological complaints. Some types of inherited eye disease lead to blindness and relatives of patients with such conditions often seek advice concerning their risk of contracting the disease.

Recent advances in molecular biology have led to the recognition of several of the genes and genetic abnormalities associated with various eye diseases. Giant leaps have been made in genetics and molecular biology such that it is now becoming the norm to refer to an inherited condition not only by the mode of inheritance but to denote the abnormal chromosome. In some cases the disease is identified by the particular gene mutation causing it. In future it is hoped that it would be possible to indicate the particular nucleotide change in the genome for each disease.

Table 23.1. Chromosome mapping for common eye diseases

Chromosome	Eye disease
1	Retinitis pigmentosa, Coppock's cataract
2	Anterior polar cataract iris coloboma Aniridia-1
5	Treacher Collins mandibulo-facial dysostosis
7p	Goldenhar's syndrome
11	Aniridia-2 (sporadic Aniridia–Wilm's tumour)
13q	Retinoblastoma
17	Neurofibromatosis type 1 (NF1) (von Recklinghausen's disease)
22q12	Neurofibromatosis type 2 (NF2)
X chromosome	Ocular albinism
	Juvenile retinoschisis Norrie's disease Choroideremia
(Xq 28)	Colour blindness – blue cone, red cone, green cone

Examples of eye disease that have been mapped out to different chromosomes are shown in Table 23.1.

Several methods are used in molecular biology to link disease to particular gene loci. First, the chromosome associations with the particular disease are determined and then the location of the gene and ultimately the specific nucleotide associated with the gene is mapped out. Methods currently available for such studies include:

- Pedigree analysis and dosage methods, which constitute linkage analysis; these are used for diseases for which no biochemical marker is available. They are mainly for dominantly inherited disease.
- Somatic hydridisation.
- Recombinant DNA techniques are used to assign known biochemical markers. Other possible uses of recombinant DNA techniques may be the future availability of enzyme production in enzyme deficient hereditary conditions.

Eye screening in selected patients at risk of inherited disease may help detect important dominant life-threatening conditions, for example, retinoblastoma, Marfan's syndrome, neurofibromatosis and von Hippel–Lindau disease. Such screening may include prenatal/intrauterine diagnosis in order to provide informed advice to parents.

Basic Genetic Mechanisms

In order to be able to give advice about the appearance of inherited disease in future generations, it is essential to have a basic knowledge of the mechanism of genetic transmission.

The nucleus of each cell in the body contains 46 chromosomes arranged as 23 pairs. The twenty-third pair comprises the sex chromosomes (the remainder being known as autosomes). These sex chromosomes are responsible for the transmission of sex characters but also carry a number of other genes unrelated to sex. In a woman the sex chromosomes are the same length but in a man one is shorter than the other. The shorter one is known as the "Y" chromosome and the longer one, which is the same as the female sex chromosome, is the "X" chromosome. When the sperm or ova are formed in the body, the pairs of chromosomes separate and the nuclei of the gametes (i.e. sperm or ova) contain only 23 chromosomes. When fertilisation occurs the 23 chromosomes from each gamete reunite as pairs. Genetic material is thus equally provided from each parent. Genes are discoid elements arranged along the length of a chromosome and each one is known to bear special influence on the development of one or more individual characteristic. Genes are arranged in pairs on adjacent chromosomes. The two genes of the pair may be similar (homozygous) or different (heterozygous). If different, one may exert an overriding influence and is said to be dominant. The gene that is overridden is said to be recessive.

Genetic disorders can be divided into three broad groups traditionally:

- abnormalities of chromosomes – numerical or structural
- abnormalities of individual genes which are transmitted to offspring
- abnormalities involving the interplay of multiple genes and the environment.

Recently, mitochondrial inheritance has been described.

Pathological genes can carry abnormalities which are transmitted to the offspring in the same way as (other) normal characteristics. In a given individual, the abnormal gene may be recessive and masked by the other one of the pair. The individual would thus not appear to have the disease but could transmit it. The four important patterns of inheritance are:

- autosomal recessive
- autosomal dominant
- sex-linked recessive
- mitochondrial inheritance.

Autosomal Recessive Inheritance

If an abnormal recessive gene is paired with another abnormal one on the opposite chromosome, it will

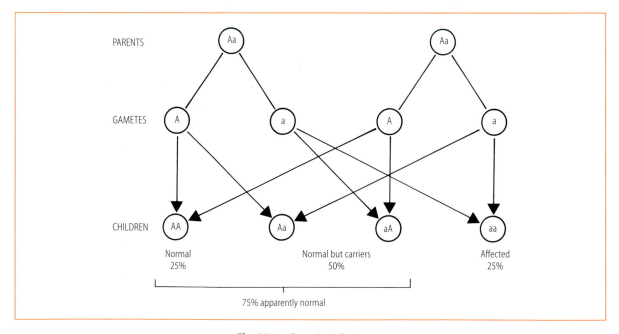

Fig. 23.1. Recessive inheritance.

have an effect, but if the opposite gene is normal, the abnormality will not become manifest. Recessive disease in clinical practice usually results from the mating of heterozygous carriers. If the abnormal gene is represented by "a", then the disease will appear in the individual with genetic configuration "aa" (homozygote) and not with the configuration "aA" (heterozygote). When two heterozygotes mate the likely offspring can be considered as in the diagram (Figure 23.1). If a patient has recessively inherited disease, his parents are likely to be normal but there may be siblings with the disease. It is important to enquire whether the parents are blood relatives because this greatly increases the likelihood of transmission. If an individual with recessive disease marries someone with the same recessive disease, then all the offspring will be affected. If one spouse is a carrier and the other has the disease then there is a risk that 50% of the offspring would be carriers and 50% would be affected. When a carrier marries a normal individual, 50% of the offspring are carriers. These expected findings could be calculated quite easily using the type of diagram shown in Figure 23.1. A common disease inherited in this manner is sickle-cell disease.

Autosomal Dominant Inheritance

When a gene bearing a defect or disease gives rise to the disease even though the other one of the pair is normal, it is said to be dominant. An affected heterozygote may therefore have 50% of affected children with a normal spouse. Of course, if both parents carry the abnormal dominant gene, then all the offspring will be affected. Dominant inheritance can only be shown with certainty if three successive generations show the disease and if about 5% of individuals are affected. Also one sex should not be affected more than the other (Figure 23.2). Examples of this type of inheritance are hereditary retinoblastoma and Marfan's disease.

Sex-linked Recessive Inheritance

It has been mentioned already that males have the "XY" configuration of sex chromosomes whereas females have "XX". Because of the unpaired nature of much of the male sex chromosomes, some recessive genes may have an effect in males when they do not do so in the female. Certain important eye conditions are carried in this way in pathological genes on the X chromosome and the pattern of inheritance is termed X-linked recessive. Examples of this type of inheritance are seen in ocular albinism and colour blindness. Retinitis pigmentosa may also show this pattern in some families. When inheritance is X-linked, only males are affected and there is no father-to-son transmission of the disease.

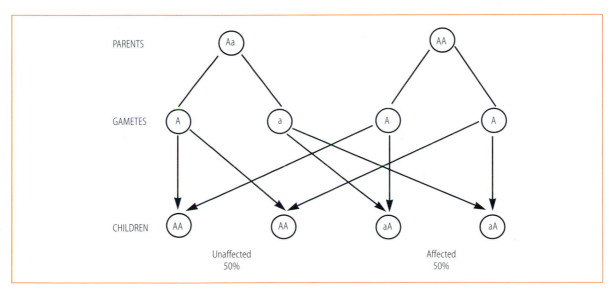

Fig. 23.2. Dominant inheritance.

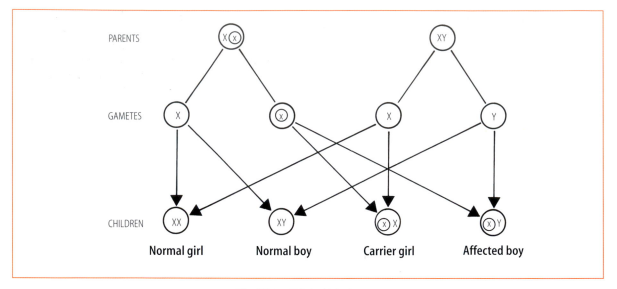

Fig. 23.3.   X-linked inheritance.

Instead it is conveyed through a carrier female to the next generation (Figure 23.3).

This description of the three important modes of inheritance should make it apparent that it is possible to predict the likely disease incidence in offspring. It should also be realised that such predictions can only be based on careful and extensive investigation of the family. Although some eye diseases are known to follow a fixed pattern of inheritance, others, notably retinitis pigmentosa, may be inherited in different ways in different families. In most large centres, genetic clinics are now in existence in which time is devoted specifically to the investigation of families and also to the detection of carriers.

Mitochondrial Inheritance

Human mitochondria contain DNA material – referred to by some as the circular DNA of mitochondria. It has been shown that human mitochondria are maternally inherited with very little or no contribution from the father. Some diseases are transmitted through the mitochondrial (or cytoplasmic) DNA. Typical examples of such transmissions are found in Leber's hereditory optic neuropathy (LHON) and chronic progressive external ophthalmoplegia (CPEO).

Chromosomal Abnormalities

Microscopic studies of the chromosomes themselves have revealed that abnormal numbers of chromosomes may be produced by a fault at the moment of fertilisation. These may be due to changes in numbers or structure of chromosomes. Numerical chromosomal changes include the absence of a chromosome (monosomy), such as in Turner's syndrome or an additional chromosome (trisomy) as in Down's syndrome. In Down's syndrome, cytogenetic studies have shown that these patients have an additional chromosome, which is indistinguishable from chromosome 21. Down's syndrome is more common in children born to older women and the eye changes include narrow palpebral fissures with a characteristic slant, cataract, high myopia and rather intriguing grey spots on the iris known as Brushfield's spots. Brushfield's spots are sometimes seen in otherwise normal individuals. Turner's syndrome (one missing X chromosome) and Klinefelter's syndrome (an extra X chromosome) are further examples of disease in which there are known to be abnormalities of the chromosome which are visible under the microscope. People with these last two diseases are of interest to the ophthalmologist on account of the abnormal but predictable manner in which they inherit colour blindness.

Structural abnormalities occur when recombination or reconstitution in an altered form follows chromosomal breaks. Such changes may be in the form of deletions, duplication inversions, translocations or isochromosomes.

Multifactorial Diseases

These are disorders that arise from an interplay of genetic and environmental influences. The genetic contribution is made up of at least two abnormal genes acting in concert to express a "dosage related" type effect, which is significantly influenced by several environmental factors. This leads to variable phenotypic expression. Examples include diabetes mellitus and some malignancies.

Drugs and the Eye 24

It is possible to achieve a high concentration of many drugs in the eye by applying them as eye drops. In this way, a high local concentration can be reached with minimal risk of systemic side-effects. The systemic side-effects of drops can be underestimated. For example, one drop of timolol can slow the pulse rate and pilocarpine drops can cause sweating and nausea. The action of local applications may be prolonged by incorporating them in an ointment but for most purposes drops are supplied in 5 or 10 ml containers. After the container has been opened it should not be kept for longer than a month. In order to avoid undue stinging, drops may be buffered to near the pH of tears and they contain a preservative such as phenyl mercuric nitrate or benzalconium chloride. It must be kept in mind that patients who develop an allergic reaction to drops may be reacting to the preservative. Single application containers are also used which do not contain a preservative.

Eye lotions are usually prescribed in 200 ml quantities and are used to irrigate the conjunctival sac. Sodium chloride eye lotion is used in first-aid to flush out foreign bodies or irritant chemicals. Fresh tapwater is an adequate substitute. Antibiotics and steroids are sometimes administered by subconjunctival injection. This is a good way of achieving high concentrations in the eye but because only 1 ml can be given at a time, the drug must be sufficiently soluble to be contained in this dose. When an eye becomes infected it is usual to give systemic as well as local antibiotics.

Treatment of Infection

Chloramphenical is rarely used as a systemic drug but it has been useful for many years in the form of eyedrops. It remains a drug of choice in this country for superficial eye infections. Other broad spectrum antibiotics in use include gentamycin, framycetin and neomycin as well as ciprofloxacin and ofloxacin. When an infection of the eye is suspected, a culture is taken from the conjunctival sac and treatment started with a wide spectrum antibiotic. Systemic and subconjunctival administration may be needed if the infection is intraocular. A number of antiviral drugs are now available but acyclovir in the form of zovirax ointment is widely used for the treatment of herpes simplex keratitis. The use of systemic acyclovir for herpes zoster has made a great impact on the severity of ocular complications.

Drops which Widen the Pupil

Routine mydriasis to allow examination of the fundus is best achieved by tropicamide 0.5% drops. They last for about 3 h. Cyclopentolate 1% can last for 24 h, but because of its cycloplegic effect is preferable for the examination of children's eyes when refraction is also needed. Dilating the pupil runs the risk of inducing an attack of acute narrow angle glaucoma in a predisposed individual. Since the vision may remain blurred driving should be avoided within the first 2 h after mydriasis. Atropine in drop form is a long-acting mydriatic, which is used when it is necessary to prevent or breakdown adhesions between iris and lens in acute iritis. It is also used in the treatment of amblyopia in children. Its effect lasts for about seven days. Allergic reactions are quite common and occasionally systemic absorption may cause central nervous system symptoms of atropine toxicity.

Drops which Constrict the Pupil

Miotics have in the past been widely used for the treatment of chronic glaucoma. Pilocarpine is available in 1%, 2%, 3% or 4% solutions. Although it is effective in reducing the intraocular pressure, the side-effects of dimming of vision and accommodation spasm can be very disabling and this treatment has largely been superseded. Pilocarpine is still used in the treatment of acute glaucoma attacks. Sometimes it is necessary to constrict the pupil rapidly during the course of intraocular surgery and this is achieved by instilling acetylcholine directly into the anterior chamber. Strong miotics run the risk of causing retinal detachment in susceptible individuals. Miotics have been used to reverse the effect of mydriatic drops used for fundus examination, but this practice is no longer recommended as a routine because it is unnecessary and the symptoms of meiosis may make matters worse.

Drugs in the Treatment of Open Angle Glaucoma

There has been a small revolution involving the type of eye drops used for the treatment of glaucoma in recent times. For years the mainstay of treatment was pilocarpine but over the past 10 years the β-blocker timolol has gradually taken its place. The systemic side-effects of this β-blocker, in particular the excacerbation of asthma, have led to the introduction of other types of ocular hypotensive agent. In general, they can be divided into cholinergic, adrenergic, prostaglandins and carbonic anhydrase inhibitors. Acetazolamide was introduced as a diuretic many years ago but although not a very good diuretic it has proved to be a potent ocular hypotensive when given orally. Again because of side-effects its use has been restricted to short-term treatment. In 1995 Dorzolamide was introduced. This is also a carbonic anhydrase inhibitor but it is available in drop form. The prostaglandin Latanoprost is beginning to prove itself as effective treatment when given as once daily drops and β-blockers other than timolol are being introduced. Adrenaline itself lowers the intraocular pressure when administered in drop form although the slight dilatation of the pupil that it causes introduced the risk of inducing narrow angle glaucoma in the predisposed.

All these medications have the problem of compliance. Elderly patients may forget to instil drops on a regular basis. The only sure way of lowering the pressure in many patients is by glaucoma surgery and many surgeons see this as a first line of treatment in some patients with open angle glaucoma.

Drugs in the Treatment of Narrow Angle Glaucoma

Narrow angle glaucoma is a surgical problem. Once the acute attack has been aborted by the use of intensive pilocarpine drops and diamox, then a small hole is made in the iris with the YAG laser and in many patients this provides a permanent cure. β-Blockers may also be used during the acute stage and more recently the α_2-agonist apraclonidine has been shown to be a useful adjunct.

Local Anaesthesia in Ophthalmology

Proxymetacaine (Ophthaine) is a useful short-acting anaesthetic drop that is comfortable to instil. Amethocaine is widely used but is longer acting and stings quite markedly. Cocaine drops are still used when carrying out surgery to the eye under local anaesthesia and the effect may last up to an hour. Local anaesthetic drops should not be used as pain relievers on a long-term basis because the anaesthetised cornea becomes ulcerated and severe infection of the eye may occur. Lignocaine with or without adrenaline is injected into the eyelids for lid surgery. Local anaesthesia for intraocular surgery is obtained by periorbital injection or sometimes retrobulbar injection of lignocaine, and for a longer effect this is sometimes combined with marcaine.

Drugs and Contact Lenses

As a rule, contact lenses should not be worn when the eye is being treated with drops. The exception is when the contact lenses themselves are being used for some therapeutic purpose. Soft hydrophilic contact lenses may take up and store the preservative from some kinds of drop. The preservative benzalkonium chloride is especially liable to be absorbed onto a contact lens. When it is essential that drops are administered to a patient wearing contact lenses, it is often possible to prescribe in the form of single dose containers which do not contain a preservative.

Artificial Tears

Artificial tears provide one of a number of measures that are used to treat tear deficiency. Other measures include occlusion of the lacrimal puncta or the use of mucolytic agents. The first step is to make the diagnosis. Once a deficiency of tears has been confirmed then the mainstay of treatment is hypromellose. Adsorptive polymers of acrylic acid can also give symptomatic relief. Polyvinyl alcohol is another compound present in a number of tear substitutes. By their nature tear substitutes tend to remain on the surface of the eye and in the conjunctival sac. For this reason their prolonged use is liable to give rise to preservative reactions. Preservative free preparations are often preferable. Some patients with a severe dry eye problem may need to instil the drops every hour or even more frequently.

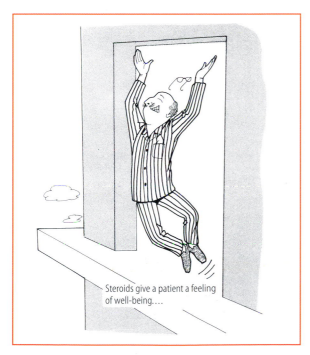

Steroids give a patient a feeling of well-being....

Fig. 24.1. There may be a false impression of the real benefit obtained.

Steroids and the Eye

Local steroids are widely used in the treatment of eye disease; systemic steroids are not used unless the sight of the eye is threatened. It must be remembered that systemic steroids give the patient a sense of well-being which may give a false impression of the real benefit obtained. Furthermore systemic steroids can have serious and life-threatening side-effects such as vertebral collapse through osteoporosis, and perforated gastric ulcer (Figure 24.1).

Local steroids should also be applied with caution, and it is a good rule always to have a specific reason for giving them. That is to say, they should not be prescribed just to make red eyes turn white without a clear diagnosis. The reasons for this are twofold: first, local steroids enhance the multiplication of viruses, especially herpes simplex; secondly, they can cause glaucoma in certain predisposed individuals. In such individuals, the instillation of one drop of steroid may cause a temporary rise of intraocular pressure. The most potent steroid in this respect is dexamethasone followed by betamethasone, prednisolone and hydrocortisone. It has been claimed that clobetasone and fluorometholone are relatively safe in this respect.

Damage to the Eyes by Drugs Administered Systemically

There are a number of drugs, which if given in excessive doses, can lead to severe visual handicap and blindness. Some of these are still available on prescription. Chloroquine and hydroxychloroquine in excessive doses can lead to pigmentary degeneration of the retina and blindness. Certain antipsychotic drugs may also cause fundus pigmentation in excessive doses; melleril and chlorpromazine have been incriminated in this respect in the past. Apart from causing glaucoma in some patients, systemic steroids are thought to increase the rate of formation of cataracts. Ethambutol may cause retinal oedema and optic atrophy. Sometimes excessive doses of quinine are taken as an abortifacient and as the patients regain consciousness they are found to be blind from quinine toxicity. Methanol is toxic to the ganglion cells of the retina and blindness is a hazard of methylated-spirit drinkers. It sometimes contaminates crudely prepared alcoholic beverages leading to unexpected loss of vision. The list of drugs with ocular side-effects is large and the reader should consult a specialised textbook for more information. Nowadays disasters and indeed law-suits should be avoidable if the drug literature is checked before prescribing an unfamiliar drug.

Section V
Blindness

Blindness 25

Blindness marks the failure or inefficacy of ophthalmological treatment. Once a patient becomes permanently blind, he or she may be lost from the care of the ophthalmologist. This means that the ophthalmologist may not have personal experience of the size of the problem and may not be in a position to experience the relative incidences of different causes of blindness. The keeping of accurate statistics is of great importance, and in order to keep statistical records it is necessary to have a clear definition of blindness. Many people who dread blindness imagine having no perception of light in each eye. Fortunately this situation is uncommon, but many people are severely debilitated by visual loss.

In the UK the major problem is among the elderly where visual loss is often combined with defective hearing. Sensory deprivation is thus a major scourge at the present time, the problem is undoubtedly going to be much worse as the proportion of elderly people increases.

Definition

In the UK the statutory definition of blindness refers to persons who "are so blind as to be unable to perform any work for which eyesight is essential". When a patient's vision falls below this level then registration as a blind person can be considered. This is a voluntary process, which allows the patient access to the social services for the visually handicapped as well as certain tax concessions. Registration is usually initiated in the hospital clinic. Some patients are referred by their general practitioners or social workers for registration by the ophthalmic specialist. A special form is completed and copies go to the patient, the general practitioner, the social services department and the Office of Population and Censuses.

Certain guidelines are laid down when considering blind registration; the visual acuity should be less than 3/60 in the worse eye but if the field of vision is very constricted then the visual acuity may be better than this. Patients whose vision is not bad enough for blind registration but none the less have significant visual handicap can have their name placed on the partially sighted register. In these patients the binocular vision should normally be worse than 6/18. Patients sometimes erroneously claim the benefits of the partially sighted because they have only one eye, even though the other eye is normal. When the vision with one or both eyes is 6/18 or better, the patient is not usually considered to be partially sighted. When one eye is completely lost through injury or disease, then the amount of incapacity is set for medico-legal purposes at about 10%. In actual fact the amount of incapacity depends a great deal on the age of the patient. A child may adapt to a remarkable degree to being one eyed, even to the extent of being able to perform with skill at ball games. Adults who become one eyed find difficulty in judging distances or performing fine manual tasks. More importantly, a number of occupations are specifically barred to those whose vision is poor in one eye.

State Benefits for the Visually Handicapped

There is no blind pension in this country but those registered blind have a special income tax allowance and some exemptions from deductions from income support. Blind persons can have parking concessions and a free National Health Service sight test as well as rail cards and bus passes. Disability living allowance may be available for blind people under the age of 65 years but for the over 65s only those both blind and deaf can qualify. Those seeking these concessions should consult an expert in the field. There are a number of voluntary organisations that run clubs, social centres and supply various other aids and benefits. For example, the Royal National Institute for the Blind (RNIB) provides a comprehensive range of services including the popular talking book service. They also supply regular funds for research into the causes of blindness.

The system of registration applies equally to children. In this instance, registration calls attention to the need for special educational requirements. These can include a specialist resource teacher, low visual aids, and other special supplies and equipment. If necessary, special schooling may need to be considered.

Standards of Vision for Various Occupations

The standards for various occupations can vary from year to year and are more or less exacting, depending on the occupation. In the UK, in order to drive a private motor vehicle, one must be able, in good daylight, to read a number plate with glasses or contact lenses at 67 feet or 20.5 metres. A full binocular field of vision is also now required. This must extend at least 120° horizontally and 20° above and below. The field is measured by perimetry using a standard target. It is assumed that any healthy person applying to drive has a normal field of vision but if the driver has any eye condition that might lead to visual handicap then he or she must declare it. The driver and vehicle licensing centre may then ask for a report from an ophthalmologist. Double vision is a bar to driving, if it cannot be corrected by prisms in the glasses or the wearing of an eye patch.

Colour Blindness

This is not blindness in any sense of the word and indeed some colour blind individuals are unaware of any problem until their colour vision is tested. Eight per cent of the male population suffers from some form of congenital colour blindness. This is usually in the form of "red-green blindness'. Inheritance of this type of defect is sex-linked so that unaffected

female carriers pass the gene to 50% of their sons. The screening of school children for colour blindness is now widely practised because of the occupational implications. The Ishihara test is the simplest and the best test for congenital colour blindness. Occupations which entail the reading of coloured warning lights or the matching of colours usually demand some form of colour vision test on entry. It is an advantage to the child to be aware of any defect during the early years of schooling.

Incidence and Cause of Blindness

In England and Wales the prevalence of blindness in 1980 for children under five years of age was 9:100,000. This figure increased to 2324:100,000 for adults over 75 years. In the west blindness in children is largely due to inherited genetic disease and birth trauma. In adults aged 20–60 years the major causes are diseases of the retina including diabetic retinopathy and optic atrophy. Over the age of 60 years macular degeneration, glaucoma and cataract are the important problems.

In Africa and Asia, the causes of blindness are rather different; many children become blind from corneal scarring associated with vitamin A deficiency and measles. Cataract is the most important cause in adults but in certain areas, for example southern Sudan, onchocerciasis and trachoma are still a serious problem.

It is apparent that the problems of blindness in Europe and North America are very different from those in poorer parts of the world where much could still be done by improving standards of nutrition and living conditions.

Aids for the Blind

The most widely recognised aid and symbol of blindness is the white stick. It is also one of the most useful aids because it identifies the patient as blind and encourages others to give assistance. Many blind people are concerned that they appear ill mannered when failing to recognise someone and are grateful for some indication of their handicap. Many different electronic devices have been tried, but by and large these are only useful to younger patients who can make full use of them. Scanning systems are now available which when moved across a book can read out a page. Most blind patients are unable to afford this type of aid. Many of these devices rely on the patients hearing to identify an audible warning signal, but most blind people prefer to use their undistracted sense of hearing as an important clue to their whereabouts. Guide dogs are specially trained by the Guide Dogs for the Blind Society and the patient must also take part in the training. Some young people find that a guide dog can expand their mobility to a great degree. Certain tactile aids are also useful, the best known of which is Braille. This system of reading for the blind was introduced from France more than 100 years ago. The letters of the alphabet are represented by numbers of raised dots on stiff paper. Blind children can learn Braille very rapidly and develop a high reading speed. Some adults find that their fingers are not sufficiently sensitive and this applies especially to diabetics. Books in Braille are now available in many different languages. Tape recordings of books and newspapers are now are now very popular amongst blind and partially sighted of all ages. The Talking Book Service provides a comprehensive library for the use of the visually disabled.

There are numerous other gadgets, which can be helpful to the blind and partially sighted; a popular one is the device that can indicate whether a teacup is full or not. For those with some residual vision, a special telephone pad with large numbers on it can be very helpful. Other ingenious devices range from relief maps which can be felt by the blind person to a telephone which speaks back through the earpiece the digit that has just been pressed. Research has also been carried out on aids that signal the position of objects by means of electrical stimuli to the skin and even by means of implanted electrodes in the visual cortex.

When the patient has a visual acuity of better than 6/60, then much can be achieved by the use of optical magnification. An ordinary hand-magnifying glass is the simplest and may often be the most effective form of assistance. If this is not adequate and the patient has been a keen reader, then a telescopic lens may be fitted to a spectacle frame with advantage. These multi-lens systems are known as low visual aids and hence the popular "LVA" clinics in eye departments for the testing and provision of these items. Apart from special telescopic lenses, closed circuit television aids are now available: a small television camera is held over the page and a magnified view of the written material is presented on a television screen.

The well-being of a blind or partially sighted person may be greatly enhanced by relatively simple social measures. Advice in the home about the use of gas or electricity may be important and the patient can be made aware of the availability of local social clubs for the blind or keep-fit classes and bus outings. An elderly patient who plays the piano may be helped by the provision of an enlarged photocopy of a favourite piece of music. In spite of all these various possibilities, one must not forget that the simplest and most useful reading aid for a partially sighted person is a good light directed on the page.

Artificial Eyes

These may be made of glass or plastic moulded to the shape of the eye socket and painted to match the other eye. Usually they are removed and washed at night by the patient and replaced the following morning. A slight degree of discharge from the socket is the rule but excessive discharge may indicate that the socket is becoming infected. This in turn may be due to roughening of the artificial eye with wear. Under these circumstances arrangements should be made for the prosthesis to be replaced or polished. It should always be borne in mind that a patient with an artificial eye may have had the eye removed because it contained a malignant tumour, in which case one must consider the possibility of local or systemic spread of the tumour. A well-made artificial eye is almost undetectable to the untrained eye but normal movements of the eye may be restricted. Nowadays the use of orbital prostheses deep to the conjunctiva and attached to the eye muscles gives greatly increased movement. After many years and after renewing the artificial eye on several occasions the eye may appear to sink downwards.

Surgical removal of an eye (enucleation) is considered in the following circumstances:

- when the eye is blind and painful
- when the eye contains a malignant tumour
- when the eye is nearly blind and sympathetic ophthalmitis is a risk following a perforating injury.

Before having an eye removed, the patient must be made fully aware of all the advantages and disadvantages. A general anaesthetic is needed and the patient remains in hospital for one or two nights after the operation. It is common practice to fit the socket with a transparent plastic "shell" for a few weeks until the artificial eye is fitted.

Further Reading

Bron A. J., Tripathi R., Watwick R., Marshall J. *Wolff's anatomy of the eye and orbit*, 8th edn. London: Chapman & Hall, 1997.

Hamilton A. M. P., Gregson R., Fish G. E. *Text atlas of the retina*. London: Martin Dunitz, 1998.

Tasman W., Jaeger E. A., Parks M. M., Benson W. E. *Duane's clinical ophthalmology* [six volumes]. Philadelphia, PA: Lippincott-Raven, 1997.

Kanski J. J. *Clinical ophthalmology*, 3rd edn. Oxford: Butterworth-Heinemann, 1997.

Index